AIDS

The U.S. Public Health Service (PHS) has been at the forefront of the AIDS battle from the beginning. The Centers for Disease Control (CDC) in Atlanta, Georgia, publishes the Morbidity and Mortality Weekly Report (MMWR) which provides the most current and in-depth accounting of the AIDS epidemic as well as reporting on individual cases. The CDC has periodically compiled all the MMWR articles dealing with AIDS into concise volumes, titled Reports on AIDS. These Reports give a national and international overview of AIDS from 1981 to the present. The CDC also publishes supplements to the MMWR targeted at specific segments of the population such as health care workers or those developing curricula on AIDS for school children. One of the most helpful supplements for information on the prevalence of AIDS and HIV infection is Human Immunodeficiency Virus Infection in the United States: A Review of Current Knowledge (Atlanta, GA, December 1987). The CDC also makes available the AIDS Weekly Surveillance Report, which details the transmission categories, risk factor combinations, and demographics of reported AIDS cases.

The National Center for Health Statistics, a division of PHS publishes the findings from the National Health Interview Survey. The most recent findings, "AIDS Knowledge and Attitudes for December 1987," published in Advance Data (Hyattsville, MD, May 1988). The results of this ongoing survey will be published in subsequent issues to describe changes in AIDS knowledge and attitudes over specific periods of time.

The U.S. Surgeon General, who heads the U.S. Public Health Service, has prepared several publications alerting the public to the dangers of AIDS. One, the Surgeon General's Report on Acquired Immune Deficiency Syndrome (WDC, 1986) contains very direct language on the transmission of AIDS and how to avoid infection. The most recent, Understanding AIDS, was sent to every American household in 1988. The Public Health Service has issued a multi-volume series, AIDS: A Public Health Challenge (WDC, 1987). Volume I, "Assessing the Problem," was most helpful in preparing this Information Plus edition.

The National Institute of Justice (NIJ), a division of the U.S. Department of Justice, has published several studies dealing with AIDS. The NIJ periodically issues "AIDS Bulletins" with warnings about risks and precautionary measures for personnel in criminal justice areas. This agency is also concerned with AIDS in correctional settings and has several updated versions of AIDS in Correctional Facilities: Issues and Options (WDC, 1987).

The Institute of Medicine of the National Academy of Sciences' Confronting AIDS: Directions for Public Health, Health Care, and Research (WDC, 1986) describes what was known about AIDS up until that date. The National Academy Press' Confronting AIDS: Update 1988 (WDC, 1988), provides a more recent assessment of the nation's progress against AIDS. Both publications provide excellent background.

The Congressional Research Service (CRS), the research arm of the Library of Congress, has published numerous "Issue Briefs" on AIDS. Acquired Immune Deficiency Syndrome and Military Manpower Policy (WDC, 1988) and Federal Funding for AIDS Research and Education provide useful facts and figures. The Office of Technology Assessment (OTA), another agency which studies current issues, has prepared several staff papers on AIDS-related issues. AIDS and Health Insurance (WDC, 1988), reports the results of an OTA survey of commercial insurers and their reactions to the epidemic.

In 1987, President Ronald Reagan appointed a task force to study various AIDS issues and offer its recommendations within a year. The final draft of the commision recommendations is the Report of The Presidential Commission on the Human Immunodeficiency Virus Epidemic (WDC, 1988). It is must reading for anyone concerned about the government's future role in dealing with the epidemic. The Global Programme (formerly the Special Programme on AIDS of the World Health Organization (WHO)) addresses the worldwide implications of this epidemic. WHO regularly publishes statistics as reported by member countries as well as articles by international experts in its monthly World Health.

The Gallup Organization, Inc., publisher of the Gallup Polls, makes its findings available monthly in the Gallup Report. We would like to thank the Gallup Organization, Inc. for permission to publish their findings on AIDS, persons with AIDS, and premarital sex. Dr. David M. Herold, of the Georgia Institute of Technology, Center for Work Performance Problems, kindly granted Information Plus permission to use information from Employees' Reactions to AIDS in the Workplace. Information Plus would also like to thank the Journal of the American Medical Association (JAMA) and officials of the Centers for Disease Control and San Francisco General Hospital for permission to print information from "Epidemiology of AIDS in Women in the United States: 1981 through 1986," by Drs. Guinan and Hardy (JAMA April 17, 1987) and "Preventing the Heterosexual Spread of AIDS," by Drs. Hearst and Hulley (JAMA April 22/29, 1988).

INFORMATION PLUS
WYLIE, TEXAS 75098
©1988
ALL RIGHTS RESERVED

EDITORS:
CAROL D. FOSTER, B.A., M.L.S.
MARK A. SIEGEL, M.A., Ph.D.
DIANA K. CHURCH, B.A., M.A.

CHAPTER I

THE NATURE OF AIDS

Acquired immune deficiency syndrome (AIDS) was identified as a new disease in 1981. By January 1988, almost 51,000 cases of AIDS, resulting in 28,500 known deaths, had been reported in the United States. The Public Health Service estimates that 1.0-1.5 million Americans are currently infected with the AIDS virus, and projects 260,000 cumulative cases of AIDS by 1991, with more than 179,000 cumulative deaths. Many consider AIDS, from which no one has recovered, the modern-day plague.

It has begun to alter the demographic makeup of New York City and San Francisco. AIDS is now the leading cause of death for men aged 25 to 44 in New York City and women aged 25 to 34. The Centers for Disease Control (CDC) reports that in 1986, AIDS was the eighth leading cause of years of potential life lost before the age of 65 in the U.S. One of every 66 babies born in New York City between November 1987 and February 1988 tested positive for HIV antibodies. In San Francisco, about half of the male homosexual population is believed to be infected with the virus, which foreshadows a huge loss of the city's population. In 1986, 40 percent of all AIDS cases occurred in New York City and San Francisco; by 1991, these two cities are expected to account for less than 20 percent, meaning the disease is expected to spread and other metropolitan areas will suffer similar economic and demographic catastrophes.

THE AIDS VIRUS

AIDS is caused by a virus which weakens the victim's immune system. A virus is a tiny infectious agent composed of genes that are surrounded by a protective coating. Viruses are parasites in that they need to invade other cells in order to reproduce. The invaded cells serve as their own death chamber because so many copies of the virus are reproduced that the cells themselves are destroyed and the host (the human) becomes diseased. The AIDS virus belongs to a special group of viruses called retroviruses, which have a special enzyme that reverses the usual pattern for translating the genetic message. Instead of going from DNA (deoxyribonucleic acid - the chemical composition of genes in living cells) to RNA (ribonucleic acid - a chemical important for cell functions), retroviruses work in reverse. The first known human retrovirus, human T-cell leukemia virus type I (HTLV-I) was discovered in 1980 by Dr. Robert Gallo and his colleagues at the U.S. National Cancer Institute.

Identifying the Virus

In September 1983, Dr. Luc Montagnier and other researchers at the Pasteur Institute in Paris, working independently of their American counter-

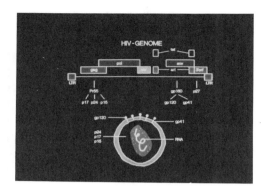

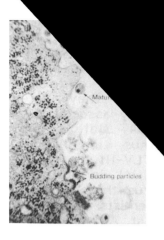

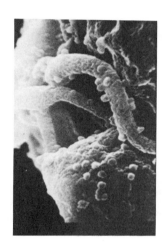

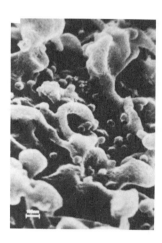

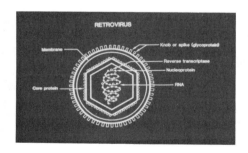

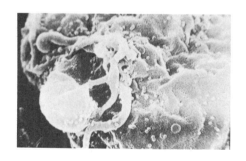

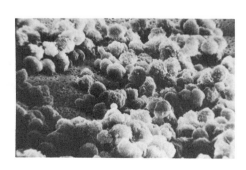

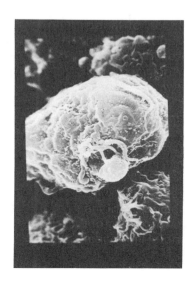

...ancer Institute, ... a retrovirus ...led lymphadeo-... LAV. In May ...lated the same ...ts, calling it ...deficiency virus ... name for the ... In 1986, French ... AIDS virus in ... The molecu-... ...ructure of HIV-II differs from HTLV-III and LAV-I, so that tests designed to detect the earlier viruses do not reveal the presence of HIV-II antibodies. The new virus, HIV-II, seems to be closely related to a virus which causes AIDS in macque monkeys. The HIV-II virus was detected in the United States for the first time in January 1988 in a woman in Newark, N.J.

HOW THE VIRUS ATTACKS THE IMMUNE SYSTEM

The AIDS virus, with seven types of genes, has proven to be more complex than most other retroviruses which have only three or four genes. Most scientists believe these genes direct protein production that make up parts of the virus and

1. Virus enters white blood cells.

2. Virus attacks T cells and multiplies.

3. T cell no longer stimulates (cellular) defense response.

4. Immune system weakened.

5. Body susceptible to "opportunistic diseases."

Source: Surgeon General's Report on Acquired Immune Deficiency Syndrome (Summary), U.S. Department of Health and Human Services, (n.d.)

regulate its reproduction. The core of the AIDS virus contains genes which are protected by a protein shell, while the entire virus is surrounded by a fatty membrane dotted with glycoproteins, or protein with sugar units attached.

White Blood Cells at Work

The immune system is a complicated, coordinated system of organs and cells, primarily various types of white blood cells which work together to prevent invasion by foreign substances. There are five types of these cells - the macrophage, T4 cell, T8 cell, plasma B cell, and the memory B cell. The macrophage, which begins as a smaller monocyte (single cell), readies the T4 cells to respond to particular invaders, i.e., a virus. At the time of attack, the macrophage, also called the vacuum cleaner of the immune system, devours the virus, but leaves a portion displayed so that the T4 cell can make contact. In addition, the macrophage stimulates reproduction of the T4 cells, resulting in thousands of T4 cells, all eager to battle the invader.

When the T4 cells attack the invading virus, they also send out chemical messages which cause the multiplication of B cells and T8 "killer" cells. These "killer" cells, with the help of some T4 cells, destroy the infected cell. Other T4 cells, which are not actively involved in destroying the infected cells, send chemical messages to B cells, causing them to reproduce and divide into groups of either plasma cells or memory cells. Plasma cells make antibodies that cripple the invading virus. Memory cells increase the immune response in case the invader ever attacks again.

Infection of the T4 Cells

Due to the complex structure of the AIDS virus, the immune system is unable to produce sufficient antibodies to fight it off. The virus attaches to the surface of the T4 molecules, the most vital link in the immune system, sheds its protective protein coat and allows its genetic material, in this case RNA, to enter the T4 cell. Reverse transcriptase, an enzyme, enters with the RNA and directs the production of DNA from the virus' RNA blueprint. The DNA then injects itself into the DNA of the T4 cell. At some later date, (it can be years later), the viral DNA can duplicate copies of the virus which then break free of the T4 cells and attack other cells. When a T4 cell has been infected, it cannot respond adequately and might reproduce as few as 10 cells instead of the 1,000 or more needed to fight the invader. When these cells do encounter the invader, the virus inside them reproduces and the cells are destroyed. To compound the situation, the AIDS virus reproduces a thousand times faster than any other known virus. The T4 cells virtually become factories for the invading enemy soldiers, producing them in overwhelming numbers.

Some T4 cells probably die as the virus particles make their way out of them. Still others die in a more sophisticated manner. Clumps of T4 cells are called syncytia. It appears that portions of the AIDS virus coat congregate on the surface of the infected cell and provide point of contact for uninfected T4 cells. These healthy cells are induced to merge with the infected cell, at which time they die. Other recent research shows the likelihood that other cells in the immune system are attacking and killing the T4 cells. The T4 cells display fragments of the AIDS virus. The T4 cells may be killed by what some scientists call an "autoimmunity" system. The AIDS virus may trick other cells in the immune system into thinking that the T4 cell is really a camouflaged AIDS virus, so the other cells do their job and kill it.

More Recent Findings

In June 1988, U.S. Army researchers, led by Dr. Monte S. Meltzer of Walter Reed Army Institute of Research in Washington, D.C., reported new findings about the nature of the AIDS virus and the macrophage. In a few rare cases, persons have been stricken with AIDS without testing positive for AIDS antibodies. Further testing beyond the normal screening found that in some cases the AIDS virus can live and reproduce within the macrophage cells without invading the T4 cells which trigger production of antibodies. This presents a continuing danger to those persons who have been exposed to the AIDS virus either through sexual activity or sharing intravenous drug syringes and who have previously tested negative.

A new method of detecting the AIDS virus, the macrophage test, though not yet generally available, may eventually replace the antibody tests (ELISA and Western blot described below) presently in use. According to Dr. Meltzer, the Army has already decided to use the new macrophage test when the other tests yield ambiguous results.

Tracking Antibodies

These findings were the result of a study of three gay men who continued to have sexual relations without a condom with persons who were known to be carriers of the AIDS virus. These men tested negative to the widely used tests for the AIDS antibodies and remained healthy. The T4 cells, which produce antibodies, were also shown to be free of the antibodies. Dr. Meltzer and his staff, however, examined the macrophages, the cells which engulf the virus and expose it to the T4 cell for the production of antibodies, and found the HIV (human immune deficiency virus) there. These men had been tracked for four to nine months and, as of June 1988, none had developed antibodies.

Several research groups have produced studies which show that everyone who has AIDS antibodies has the virus in their macrophages. The AIDS virus can live and grow in the macrophage cells until these cells are filled to the point of bursting without killing the cells, while the virus kills the T4 cells when it grows within them. Because macrophages are capable of spreading the virus through bodily fluids, persons with the virus in the macrophages are also considered infectious. At this point, it is uncertain if those with HIV only in their macrophages are as likely to develop AIDS or not. This new evidence may partially explain the delay of up to one year for the antibodies to develop in some victims; the virus could be hiding in the macrophages.

Other Viruses?

Mounting evidence suggests that the AIDS virus remains dormant until any number of other viruses trigger the disease. Perhaps a later infection activates the T4 cells. Under normal circumstances, an attack on the T4 cells is just what the doctor ordered to fight an infection. However, if the T4 cells are laden with the deadly AIDS virus, their call to action ultimately cripples the immune system. Other researchers suggest that other viruses might "turn on" the AIDS virus, even if the T4 cells are not activated. One possibility is that viruses and other agents damage the cell's DNA in some way, thereby increasing the production of the HIV. Ultraviolet rays from sunlight have been reported to increase HIV production and damage DNA.

PROGRESSION OF THE INFECTION

Once the immune system has been attacked, AIDS victims become susceptible to bacteria and cancer (opportunistic infections) that the immune system might otherwise be able to fend off if it were intact. As mentioned earlier, when the virus enters the blood and attacks the T4 cells, antibodies are formed. These antibodies can be detected in the blood by a simple test, often within two to three weeks after the infection. Even before a person tests positive, however, he or she can transmit the virus to others by methods which will be explained in the following chapter.

After the infection, several things can happen. Some infected persons remain "well", or symptom free, but are still able to infect others. Others may develop a disease less serious than AIDS, that has come to be known as AIDS Related Complex (ARC). In still others, once the protective immune system has been destroyed, other germs (bacteria, protozoa, fungi, and other viruses) and cancers use the opportunity presented by a lowered resistance to infect and destroy. One of the most common opportunistic disease is Pneumocystis carinii pneumonia, a lung infection caused by fungus and usually found in cancer and transplant patients whose immune systems are weakened. Another is Kaposi's sarcoma, a rare cancer of the blood vessel walls causing purple lesions on the skin.

CHAPTER II

DEFINITION, SYMPTOMS, AND TRANSMITTAL OF AIDS

A DEFINITION OF AIDS

The Centers for Disease Control (CDC), a division of the U.S. Public Health Service, revised its definition for AIDS effective September 1, 1987. Prior to that date, the CDC definition for AIDS included patients with a depressed immune system who had one major illness tied to the syndrome. Alternative definitions included patients with a depressed immune system, a positive AIDS antibody blood test, and one disease from a list of lesser infections. The recent, and more inclusive, definition resulted from researchers' concerns that these definitions omitted many very ill people with AIDS antibodies, who were experiencing "progressive, seriously disabling, and even fatal conditions" which were not being monitored by epidemiologists. For reporting purposes the new definition includes most of the severe non-infectious, non-cancerous HIV-associated conditions that the CDC has recognized as being associated with HIV infection among children and adults.

Without Laboratory Evidence

If laboratory tests were not performed, or the results of tests were inconclusive, and there is no other explanation for immunodeficiency (the inability of the immune system to fight off infections), then the presence of certain diseases, if diagnosed by a carefully definitive method, indicates the presence of AIDS. (CDC includes such definitive diagnostic methods as microscopy, endoscopy, autopsy, culture, and other clinical methods of investigation as definitive). Legitimate causes for immunodeficiency are high-doses or long-term systemic corticosteroid therapy; diseases such as Hodgkin's disease or other diseases involving the lymph nodes; or a congenital (genetic) immunodeficiency syndrome. If none of the causes are present, then the presence of any one of eleven different diseases, primarily various forms of cancer and pneumonia is AIDS. These causes and diseases are found in the accompanying 1987 Revision of Case Definition for AIDS. If none of the diseases in Section I.B has been definitively diagnosed, then again, there is no AIDS case. However, if one of these diseases is diagnosed and no other explanation exists for immunodeficiency, then it is considered an AIDS case.

With Laboratory Evidence

Even if other causes for immunodeficiency such as those listed in Section I.A are present, if laboratory results produce a positive result for an HIV in-

1987 REVISION OF CASE DEFINITION FOR AIDS FOR SURVEILLANCE PURPOSES

For national reporting, a case of AIDS is defined as an illness characterized by one or more of the following "indicator" diseases, depending on the status of laboratory evidence of HIV infection, as shown below.

I. Without Laboratory Evidence Regarding HIV Infection

If laboratory tests for HIV were not performed or gave inconclusive results (*See* Appendix I) and the patient had no other cause of immunodeficiency listed in Section I.A below, then any disease listed in Section I.B indicates AIDS if it was diagnosed by a definitive method (*See* Appendix II).

A. Causes of immunodeficiency that disqualify diseases as indicators of AIDS in the absence of laboratory evidence for HIV infection

1. high-dose or long-term systemic corticosteroid therapy or other immuno-suppressive/cytotoxic therapy ≤3 months before the onset of the indicator disease

2. any of the following diseases diagnosed ≤3 months after diagnosis of the indicator disease: Hodgkin's disease, non-Hodgkin's lymphoma (other than primary brain lymphoma), lymphocytic leukemia, multiple myeloma, any other cancer of lymphoreticular or histiocytic tissue, or angioimmunoblastic lymphadenopathy

3. a genetic (congenital) immunodeficiency syndrome or an acquired immunodeficiency syndrome atypical of HIV infection, such as one involving hypogammaglobulinemia

B. Indicator diseases diagnosed definitively (*See* Appendix II)

1. candidiasis of the esophagus, trachea, bronchi, or lungs
2. cryptococcosis, extrapulmonary
3. cryptosporidiosis with diarrhea persisting >1 month
4. cytomegalovirus disease of an organ other than liver, spleen, or lymph nodes in a patient >1 month of age
5. herpes simplex virus infection causing a mucocutaneous ulcer that persists longer than 1 month; or bronchitis, pneumonitis, or esophagitis for any duration affecting a patient >1 month of age
6. Kaposi's sarcoma affecting a patient < 60 years of age
7. lymphoma of the brain (primary) affecting a patient < 60 years of age
8. lymphoid interstitial pneumonia and/or pulmonary lymphoid hyperplasia (LIP/PLH complex) affecting a child <13 years of age
9. *Mycobacterium avium* complex or *M. kansasii* disease, disseminated (at a site other than or in addition to lungs, skin, or cervical or hilar lymph nodes)
10. *Pneumocystis carinii* pneumonia
11. progressive multifocal leukoencephalopathy
12. toxoplasmosis of the brain affecting a patient >1 month of age

II. With Laboratory Evidence for HIV Infection

Regardless of the presence of other causes of immunodeficiency (I.A), in the presence of laboratory evidence for HIV infection (*See* Appendix I), any disease listed above (I.B) or below (II.A or II.B) indicates a diagnosis of AIDS.

A. Indicator diseases diagnosed definitively (*See* Appendix II)

1. bacterial infections, multiple or recurrent (any combination of at least two within a 2-year period), of the following types affecting a child < 13 years of age:

   septicemia, pneumonia, meningitis, bone or joint infection, or abscess of an internal organ or body cavity (excluding otitis media or superficial skin or mucosal abscesses), caused by *Haemophilus*, *Streptococcus* (including pneumococcus), or other pyogenic bacteria

2. coccidioidomycosis, disseminated (at a site other than or in addition to lungs or cervical or hilar lymph nodes)

3. HIV encephalitis (also called "HIV dementia," "AIDS dementia," or "subacute encephalitis due to HIV") (*See* Appendix II for description)

4. histoplasmosis, disseminated (at a site other than or in addition to lungs or cervical or hilar lymph nodes)

5. isosporiasis with diarrhea persisting >1 month
6. Kaposi's sarcoma at any age
7. lymphoma of the brain (primary) at any age
8. other non-Hodgkin's lymphoma of B-cell or unknown immunologic phenotype and the following histologic types:

   a. small noncleaved lymphoma (either Burkitt or non-Burkitt type) (*See* Appendix IV for equivalent terms and numeric codes used in the *International Classification of Diseases*, Ninth Revision, Clinical Modification)

   b. immunoblastic sarcoma (equivalent to any of the following, although not necessarily all in combination: immunoblastic lymphoma, large-cell lymphoma, diffuse histiocytic lymphoma, diffuse undifferentiated lymphoma, or high-grade lymphoma) (*See* Appendix IV for equivalent terms and numeric codes used in the *International Classification of Diseases*, Ninth Revision, Clinical Modification)

   Note: Lymphomas are not included here if they are of T-cell immunologic phenotype or their histologic type is not described or is described as "lymphocytic," "lymphoblastic," "small cleaved," or "plasmacytoid lymphocytic"

9. any mycobacterial disease caused by mycobacteria other than *M. tuberculosis*, disseminated (at a site other than or in addition to lungs, skin, or cervical or hilar lymph nodes)

10. disease caused by *M. tuberculosis*, extrapulmonary (involving at least one site outside the lungs, regardless of whether there is concurrent pulmonary involvement)

11. *Salmonella* (nontyphoid) septicemia, recurrent

12. HIV wasting syndrome (emaciation, "slim disease") (*See* Appendix II for description)

B. Indicator diseases diagnosed presumptively (by a method other than those in Appendix II)

Note: Given the seriousness of diseases indicative of AIDS, it is generally important to diagnose them definitively, especially when therapy that would be used may have serious side effects or when definitive diagnosis is needed for eligibility for antiretroviral therapy. Nonetheless, in some situations, a patient's condition will not permit the performance of definitive tests. In other situations, accepted clinical practice may be to diagnose presumptively based on the presence of characteristic clinical and laboratory abnormalities. Guidelines for presumptive diagnoses are suggested in Appendix III.

1. candidiasis of the esophagus
2. cytomegalovirus retinitis with loss of vision
3. Kaposi's sarcoma
4. lymphoid interstitial pneumonia and/or pulmonary lymphoid hyperplasia (LIP/PLH complex) affecting a child <13 years of age
5. mycobacterial disease (acid-fast bacilli with species not identified by culture), disseminated (involving at least one site other than or in addition to lungs, skin, or cervical or hilar lymph nodes)
6. *Pneumocystis carinii* pneumonia
7. toxoplasmosis of the brain affecting a patient >1 month of age

III. With Laboratory Evidence Against HIV Infection

With laboratory test results negative for HIV infection (*See* Appendix I), a diagnosis of AIDS for surveillance purposes is ruled out *unless*:

A. all the other causes of immunodeficiency listed above in Section I.A are excluded; AND

B. the patient has had either:

1. *Pneumocystis carinii* pneumonia diagnosed by a definitive method (*See* Appendix II); OR

2. a. any of the other diseases indicative of AIDS listed above in Section I.B diagnosed by a definitive method (*See* Appendix III); AND

   b. a T-helper/inducer (CD4) lymphocyte count <400/mm³.

Source: "Revision of the CDC Surveillance Case Definition for Acquired Immunodeficiency Syndrome." *Morbidity and Mortality Weekly Report*, August 14, 1987.

fection, the presence of any disease listed in Section I.B or Sections II.A or II.B, indicates an AIDS diagnosis. If diseases from neither Section I.B or Section II.A, which now include such conditions as emaciation and HIV encephalitis have been definitively diagnosed, and no disease from Section II.B has been presumptively diagnosed, even with a positive test result, then there is not an AIDS case. A presumptive diagnosis, while not as preferred as a definitive diagnosis, is necessary when the patient's performance prohibits definitive tests. Then diagnosis is made based on the presence of characteristic clinical and laboratory abnormalities.

With Negative Laboratory Evidence

When laboratory test results for an HIV infection are negative, diagnosis for AIDS, for the benefit of surveillance purposes, is not ruled out unless all the other causes explaining immunodeficiency (see Section I.A) are ruled out; and the patient has either

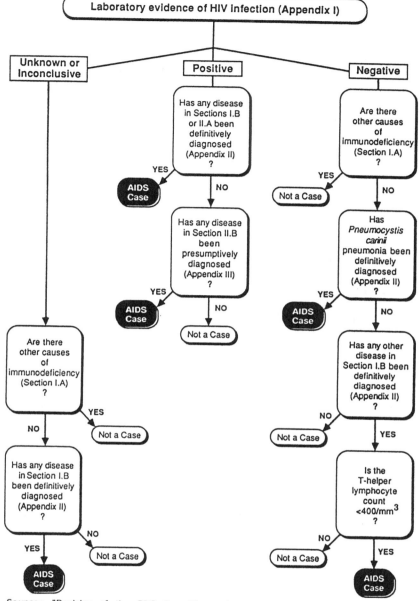

Source: "Revision of the CDC Surveillance Case Definition for Acquired Immunodeficiency Syndrome," Morbity and Mortality Weekly Report, August 14, 1987.

Pneumocystis carinii pneumonia, definitively diagnosed; or any of the other disease listed in Section I.B, definitively diagnosed; and a T-helper-inducer (CD4) lymphocyte count less than 400/mm3.

INCUBATION PERIOD

Researchers and scientists believe the incubation period of AIDS to be between 4 to 6 years, on the average. Various studies have found that 20 to 30 percent of those infected with the virus develop AIDS within five years of the infection. Many develop the less serious AIDS-Related Complex (ARC), but this is often the first stage of developing AIDS. Still others have the virus for several years with no signs or symptoms. Because the track history of this disease is short, despite the extensive research, there is no way to to determine how many, if any, infected persons will remain symptom-free.

SIGNS AND SYMPTOMS

No Signs

Some infected persons develop no physically apparent symptoms of illness. Considerable research is being done to determine why some infected persons remain healthy years after being infected while others succumb to the disease and die within months.

AIDS-Related Complex (ARC)

ARC is a condition caused by the AIDS virus in which the patient tests positive for AIDS infection and has a specific set of clinical symptoms which tend to be less severe than those of someone with AIDS. These may include loss of appetite, weight loss, fever, night sweats, skin rashes, diarrhea, tiredness, lack of resistance to infection, or swollen lymph nodes. Because these are often signs and symptoms of other diseases, a physician should be consulted.

Acquired Immune Deficiency Syndrome (AIDS)

Only a qualified health professional can diagnose AIDS. While some AIDS symptoms are similar to those described above for ARC, they are more serious and these, coupled with the opportunistic diseases such as Pneumocystis carinii and Kaposi's sarcoma, always mean the condition is fatal. These symptoms include a general malaise; weight loss; nausea; fever; night sweats; swollen lymph glands; a heavy, persistent, dry cough; easy brusability or unexplained bleeding; watery diarrhea; loss of memory; balance problems; mood changes; blurring or loss of vision; and thrush (a white coating of the tongue and throat). Very often it is the opportunistic diseases and not the AIDS virus which causes the person's death. The AIDS virus is basically the same in all infected persons – it is the reactions within each individual which vary dramatically.

INFECTED, BUT HEALTHY

While many researchers concentrate on how the AIDS HIV can cause so much harm, still others are looking at why it does not cause the same harm in everyone. In June 1987, scientists in New York were still tracking 13 gay men, who had volunteered for the hepatitis B vaccine study in 1978, and were infected with HIV at the time. In the nine years which followed, none had shown signs or symptoms of the disease. Dr. Chadd E. Stevens, the head epidemiologist at the New York Blood Center, reports that the immune systems of these 13 men look "perfectly normal".

In spite of the fact that some experts believe that all who are infected will develop the disease over a period of time, much could be learned from studying those who have remained healthy for relatively long periods of time. While there are very few known longtime carriers of the disease, evidence shows that some are advancing towards AIDS, while others are not. While all infectious diseases have a varying ratio of those who become ill to those who never develop symptoms, there are very few illnesses that kill everyone who develops the symptoms. There are also few other diseases in which those infected become lifetime carriers and can spread the infection to other people under particular circumstances. Information derived from research on those who have remained symptom-free is useful to health professionals when they are faced with advising those who become infected on their chances of developing AIDS. Such research could also be vital to government officials who must plan for the economic and social fallout from AIDS.

While most consider these explanations little more than guesswork, the following are some ideas on the difference in susceptibility among various persons.

1.   Genetics.   A team from St. Mary's Hospital and Medical School in London as well as one from the U.S. National Cancer Institute have reported links between AIDS susceptibility and various inherited blood proteins.

2.   Virulence.   Research is ongoing to determine if different strains are disproportionate in virulence (poisonousness).

3.   Habits and environment.   Epidemiologists are searching for factors such as use of certain drugs or past diseases which may separate those who do not develop AIDS from those who do.

4.   Immune differences.   A number of different groups are exploring the possibility that long-term HIV carriers, as well as those who have been exposed to the virus repeatedly without becoming infected, have something unusual or distinctive about their immune systems, such as a factor in the blood which can "neutralize" the AIDS virus.

5.   Reversibility.   Dr. Richard A. Kaslow, a leading AIDS epidemiologist at the National Institutes of Health, reports that there is unclear evidence that "a very few" people may have developed symptoms, but later recovered.

6.   Reverters.   A preliminary report for the National Institutes of Health indicates that five people from among 4,955 who originally showed evidence of antibodies to AIDS, showed no such evidence when given follow-up tests.

Differences exist between researchers in defining a "healthy" AIDS virus carrier.   Some restrict the term healthy to those who remain symptom-free and whose tests indicated that their immune system and other functions are normal. Still others have adopted a broader approach, classifying as healthy those who may have swollen lymph nodes and abnormal test results, but who continue to feel fine.   While some remain well several years after becoming infected is a signal for guarded optimism, Dr. Jaffe of the Centers for Disease Control in Atlanta calls the fact that some do become ill after so many years of being infected "sobering."   No one knows what 20 or 30 years down the line will hold.

TRANSMISSION OF AIDS

Perhaps the only thing as frightening as the knowledge of what AIDS does, is the lack of knowledge by the public of how AIDS is transmitted.   A Public Health Service advertisement reports that "The only thing spreading faster than AIDS is rumors."   The only way for this understandable fear to stop short of panic is to make the causes of AIDS known to everyone.   In the brochure, Understanding AIDS (WDC, 1988), sent to every Americans household in the Spring of 1988, Dr. C. Everett Koop, Surgeon General of the United States warns that, "Who you are has nothing to do with whether you are in danger if being infected with the AIDS virus.   What matters is what you do."   To be sure, there are "high risk groups" of people, but they are not the only ones who become infected with the AIDS virus.

Known Ways of Transmission

No proof currently exists to show that the AIDS virus is transmitted in any other way than:

1. By having oral, anal, or vagina sex with an infected person.

2. By sharing drug needles or syringes with an infected person.

3. From an infected mother to her baby at some point around the time of birth (possibly also through breast milk).

4. By receiving a transplanted organ or bodily fluids, such as blood transfusions or blood products from an infected person.

High concentrations of HIV have been found in blood, semen, and cerebro-spinal fluid. Concentrations up to 1,000 times smaller have been found in saliva, tears, vaginal secretions, breast milk, and bowel movements. While no cases have been attributed to intimate kissing, health officials advise caution and most dentists and opthamologists now wear rubber gloves.

Casual Contact

In the Surgeon General's Report on Acquired Immune Deficiency Syndrome (WDC, 1986), Dr. Koop reported that AIDS is an infectious, contagious disease, but is not spread in the same manner as a common cold or measles or chicken pox. It is not spread by common everyday contact such as sneezing or coughing by infected persons, or by sharing bathrooms or swimming pools, or hugging or shaking hands with a person with AIDS or someone who carries the virus. Studies of family members who lived with and cared for AIDS patients show no one who became infected through casual contact.

Pets and Mosquitoes

Household pets, such as dogs and cats, and other domestic animals are not a source of infection from the AIDS virus, nor are mosquitoes or other insects.

In 1985, the Centers for Disease Control in Atlanta noted an unusually dense concentration of AIDS sufferers in Belle Glade, FL, an area infested with mosquitoes. Speculation soon followed that mosquitoes might be possible trans-ports for the deadly disease as they were for malaria and yellow fever.

In June 1987, scientists in collaboration with the National Cancer Insti-tute, found that while mosquitoes could retain the AIDS virus in their bodies for two or three days after ingesting infected blood, there was no evidence that the virus could multiply inside the mosquitoes as it did in humans, or that the mosquitoes were capable of transmitting the virus once they had it. Similar studies by French scientists of African insects have yielded like findings. The fact the virus does not multiply inside the mosquito is a posi-tive sign, since larger volumes of the virus would infect the mosquito for longer periods of time, but even then, some feel it would be too little of the virus to spread the infection.

Giving and Receiving Blood

The Surgeon General reports, and other health officials agree, that there is no danger of transmitting the AIDS virus from donating blood. The needles used to draw blood from a donor are all brand-new and are discarded after they are used once. Contact with the AIDS virus from donating blood is virtually impossible.

To deny that there is no risk of AIDS from a blood transfusion would be false. The risk over the past few years has been reduced considerably since the advent of certain laboratory tests which can identify the AIDS antibody (see below). Unfortunately for many hemophiliacs, (those whose blood does not clot naturally, so blood or blood product transfusions are necessary), these tests are too little, too late. Presently, donors are screened for risk factors (homosexual behavior, IV drug use, etc.) in addition to testing blood for antibodies.

TESTING FOR AIDS

A person who has been infected with the AIDS virus produces antibodies to that virus. While these antibodies are not enough to fight the virus, they do indicate the presence of the virus. Testing is done for AIDS antibodies rather than the virus itself, because the virus is difficult to isolate from the blood. Tests have a dual purpose: they diagnose the AIDS infection, and they screen blood used in transfusions to determine their safety. A major problem with the current forms of testing is the nature of the virus. Usually antibodies appear in six to 12 weeks following the infection, but some reported cases have taken up to one year to appear. Another problem is the accuracy of the tests.

ELISA, one such test used for screening, rather than diagnosis, was made available for commercial use in May 1985. ELISA (enzyme-linked immunosorbent assay) uses antigens derived from the HIV (human immunodeficiency virus). ELISA is simple to use and inexpensive, but has been plagued by the number of false positive results it indicates. In this test, a sample of the blood to be tested is added to proteins from the AIDS virus. If antibodies are present, they will attach themselves to the virus particles. Through chemical reactions, the color of the mixture will change. Because of the test's unreliability, another test, the more sophisticated and expensive Western blot technique, is often performed to confirm the ELISA results. A positive result does not mean the person has AIDS, but that he/she does have the antibodies to the AIDS virus which indicates exposure.

The Western blot test is used by placing various AIDS proteins on a special paper strip according to size. The blood sample is then applied to the paper. If there are HIV antibodies in the blood, they will bind to the various proteins on the paper. Chemicals are added which produce bands of color wherever antibodies have adhered to viral proteins. The Western blot provides a positive, a negative, or an intermediate result. The presence of three or more of the color bands usually confirms infection with the AIDS virus. If fewer bands are present, the test is considered intermediate and retesting occurs six months later. If no color bands appear, the test is considered negative with no virus present.

In 1985, blood banks began instituting these tests on donated blood. While the nation's blood supply is probably safer than it has ever been, as a result of this testing, there is still the very real possibility that tainted blood does get past the screening process. Studies vary greatly in their estimation of the number of tainted blood units which pass the test and are erroneously considered safe. Estimates vary from 25 chances in a million units of blood received into the system, to only 4 chances per million.

13

CHAPTER III

THOSE WHO ARE AT RISK

Everyone is at risk of infection with the human immunodeficiency virus (HIV) if he or she fails to take the precautions which prevent such infection. (See Chapter XI). Some groups are high risk through no fault of their own - hemophiliacs and children born to mothers carrying the HIV. Most others are at risk because of behavior, which if modified, could considerably lower their risk. This chapter will discuss those at "high risk", those at risk within the general population, and the prevalence of infection among them.

RECOGNIZED HIGH RISK

Homosexual and Bisexual Men

The Centers for Disease Control (CDC), a division of the U.S. Public Health Service, reports that homosexual and bisexual men remain the major groups at increased risk for HIV infection. Findings from 50 surveys and studies in 22 cities and 15 states done since 1984 show prevalence rates ranging from 10 percent to as high as 70 percent, with most between 20 percent and 50 percent. With the exception of high prevalence rates among homosexual men in San Francisco, the prevalence among other homosexual men varies geographically without significant concentration in any one region.

The CDC cautions that their data may overestimate the prevalence of HIV infection among these men since most of the studies were conducted among patients at sexually transmitted disease (STD) clinics. Generally, those who require medical care at these clinics are those who put themselves at high risk through their sexual behavior. There is little comparable data on homosexual and bisexual men who are not seeking medical care, including those who may be at lower risk for infection.

---

* All current studies indicate that virtually everyone who is infected with the HIV eventually develops AIDS. According to the CDC, the incubation period presently has a median of 7 years. Bear this in mind when examining the following data on the number of reported AIDS cases. All of those who are presently infected with the virus have not yet developed AIDS, and may not develop the disease AIDS for several years. However, once they are infected, they are carriers and can transmit the virus under limited circumstances.

AIDS CASES REPORTED TO HAVE A SINGLE RISK FACTOR	Number	Percent
Homosexual/Bisexual Male	37542	(60.8)
Intravenous (IV) Drug Abuse	10107	(16.4)
Hemophilia/Coagulation Disorder	341	(0.6)
Heterosexual Contact[2]	2408	(3.9)
Transfusion, Blood/Components	1527	(2.5)
Undetermined[3]	1989	(3.2)
SUBTOTAL	53914	(87.3)

AIDS CASES REPORTED TO HAVE MULTIPLE RISK FACTORS	Number	Percent
Homosexual-Bi Male/Blood Transfusion	742	(1.2)
Homosexual-Bi Male/Heterosexual Contact	632	(1.0)
Homosexual-Bi Male/Heterosexual Contact/Blood Transfusion	31	(0.1)
Homosexual-Bi Male/Hemophilia	27	(0.0)
Homosexual-Bi Male/Hemophilia/Blood Transfusion	24	(0.0)
Homosexual-Bi Male/Hemophilia/Heterosexual Contact	2	(0.0)
Homosexual-Bi Male/Hemophilia/Heterosexual Contact/Blood Transfusion	1	(0.0)
Homosexual-Bi Male/IV Drug Abuse	4177	(6.8)
Homosexual-Bi Male/IV Drug Abuse/Blood Transfusion	136	(0.2)
Homosexual-Bi Male/IV Drug Abuse/Heterosexual Contact	225	(0.4)
Homosexual-Bi Male/IV Drug Abuse/Heterosexual Contact/Blood Transfusion	15	(0.0)
Homosexual-Bi Male/IV Drug Abuse/Hemophilia	7	(0.0)
Homosexual-Bi Male/IV Drug Abuse/Hemophilia/Blood Transfusion	7	(0.0)
Homosexual-Bi Male/IV Drug Abuse/Hemophilia/Heterosexual Contact	1	(0.0)
IV Drug Abuse/Blood Transfusion	342	(0.6)
IV Drug Abuse/Heterosexual Contact	969	(1.6)
IV Drug Abuse/Heterosexual Contact/Blood Transfusion	72	(0.1)
IV Drug Abuse/Hemophilia	16	(0.0)
IV Drug Abuse/Hemophilia/Blood Transfusion	11	(0.0)
IV Drug Abuse/Hemophilia/Heterosexual Contact	2	(0.0)
IV Drug Abuse/Hemophilia/Heterosexual Contact/Blood Transfusion	5	(0.0)
Hemophilia/Blood Transfusion	258	(0.4)
Hemophilia/Heterosexual Contact	2	(0.0)
Hemophilia/Heterosexual Contact/Blood Transfusion	5	(0.0)
Heterosexual Contact/Blood Transfusion	127	(0.2)
SUBTOTAL	7836	(12.7)
TOTAL	61750	(100.0)

[1] These data are provisional. Not all risk factors may have been determined or reported for all cases.

[2] Includes persons who have had heterosexual contact with a person with AIDS or at risk for AIDS and persons without other identified risks who were born in countries in which heterosexual transmission is believed to play a major role although precise means of transmission have not yet been fully defined.

[3] Includes patients on whom risk information is incomplete (due to death, refusal to be interviewed or loss to follow-up), patients still under investigation, men reported only to have had heterosexual contact with a prostitute, and interviewed patients for whom no specific risk was identified; also includes one health-care worker who seroconverted to HIV and developed AIDS after documented needlestick to blood.

Source: "AIDS Weekly Surveillance Report,"
Centers for Disease Control, May 23, 1988

Of the 60,623 cases of AIDS reported to CDC by May 9, 1988, 38,371 (63 percent) were homosexual or bisexual males. These men also accounted for 63 percent of the 33,960 deaths reported to CDC since June 1981. Homosexual and bisexual males represent 61 percent of AIDS cases reported to have a single risk factor. (Risk factor are those circumstances which place one at risk for infection: homosexual behavior, IV drug use, sexual relations with an infected partner, hemophilia or blood tranfusion during a certain time period.) Because this group is at the greatest risk, those who have additional risk factors, such as being hemophiliac, and/or receiving a blood transfusion, and especially if they are IV drug abusers, are in greater jeopardy than any others.

Intravenous Drug Users

The majority of intravenous (IV) drug users who tested positive for the presence of HIV antibody were located on the East Coast. In 90 studies in 53 cities in 27 states and territories, rates in New York City, northern New Jersey, and Puerto Rico ranged from 50 to 60 percent, while rates for most other areas of the country were generally below 5 percent.

As with the data on homosexual men, most of the statistics on IV drug users is obtained from clinical settings, in this case, treatment centers, which primarily treat heroin addicts. Many experts believe that those who undergo treatment represent only 15 percent of the estimated 1.1 million IV drug users in this country. Many feel that those

HIV antibody prevalence in homosexual and bisexual men, 50 surveys and studies, United States, 1984-1987

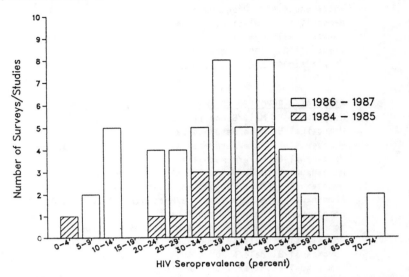

HIV antibody prevalence in IV drug users, 90 surveys and studies, United States, 1984-1987

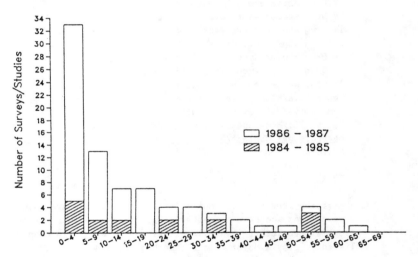

Source: "Human Immunodeficiency Virus Infection in the United States," Morbity and Mortality Weekly Report, December 18, 1987.

who are not in treatment and who are habitual users are at even greater risk for infections. At the same time, the estimated 200,000 intermittent users may have a lower prevalence of infection because of less frequent exposure to contaminated needles and equipment which transmit the infection.

While the problem of AIDS among IV drug users is especially severe in the Northeast, other areas which currently have lower prevalence rates, have the potential for substantial increases in infection as users continue to share needles and equipment. Drug abusers who carry the HIV infection can seriously affect those around them - their sex partners and children, even unborn children are also at risk. Infection caused by IV drug use has been the major source of AIDS contracted through heterosexual contact in the U.S. It is also the direct and indirect source for the great majority of perinatally (at the time of birth) acquired AIDS cases. Because so much time can pass between infection and development of AIDS, it is difficult to determine the real rate of HIV infection. Further HIV surveillance of IV drug users is necessary in order to develop effective education and risk reduction programs.

IV drug users make up 19 percent (11,256) of the cumulative number of AIDS cases and 19 percent (6,311) of the deaths reported by May 9, 1988. Homosexual males, who were also IV drug users, accounted for an additional 4,500 AIDS cases, and were 7 percent of the total cases and 8 percent of the cumulative deaths.

Hemophiliacs

Because screening for HIV antibody was not available until 1985, many hemophiliacs (persons whose blood does not clot properly) were exposed to infection with HIV. The high prevalence of persons with HIV infection with hemophilia A or B is evenly distributed across the country, a result of the national distribution of clotting factor concentrates they received before 1985. Studies show that HIV infection differs by the type and severity of the coagulation disorder. Generally, 70 percent of those persons who had hemophilia A and 35 percent with hemophilia B were positive. Since hemophilia B is usually less severe than hemophilia A, the former group needed fewer treatments with the clotting factor, and, therefore, they were exposed to HIV-contaminated products fewer times. The CDC cautions that these rates may be overrepresented, since the studies were performed at hemophilia treatment centers where patients with more severe hemophilia are likely to be found than those with a mild case of the disease.

Since the beginning of cumulative (on-going) record keeping of AIDS cases and deaths in June 1981, 597 persons with hemophilia or coagulation disorders and 1,1492 persons who received blood transfusions or components have come down with AIDs and 353 and 1,004, respectively, have died. These categories together total 4 percent of those afflicted with the disease and the same percentage of those who have died.

Heterosexual Partners of Those at Risk

Studies have been conducted among persons who are in heterosexual relationships with an HIV-infected person, and have no other identified risk factor for acquiring the infection. The prevalence rates for persons in this category range from under 10 percent to as high as 60 percent. Research has not yet determined why there are these huge differences. It is unclear if the degree of infectiousness of the source partners differs among the various risk groups. Some studies have shown that infectiousness increases as the immune system of the partner with AIDS deteriorates. Other variables include the frequency and type of sexual exposure. Anal intercourse appears to increase the possibility of infection since the vulnerable nature of the rectum lining allows the AIDS virus easy entry into the blood stream. More male-to-female than female-to-male transmission has been recorded, but data is insufficient to definitely establish a pattern.

Since not all persons who are at recognized risk - bisexual, IV drug users, and hemophiliacs - are infected, their partners should have a lower infection prevalence than partners of persons known to be infected. Limited data available on heterosexual partners of high-risk persons whose HIV status is unknown shows a lower risk, ranging from 0 to 11 percent.

Since 1981, almost 2,500 cases of AIDS have been recorded in which heterosexual contact was listed as the means of transmission. Nearly 1,500 of these persons, mostly female, were believed to have contracted AIDS due to heterosexual contact with a person with AIDS or who was at risk for AIDS. The remaining 1,000 persons were without other identified risks, but were born in countries where heterosexual activity is a major mode of transmission.

RISK AMONG THE GENERAL POPULATION

The general population is composed of persons who are at various levels of risk for HIV infection. The data compiled by CDC on select groups is biased to the degree

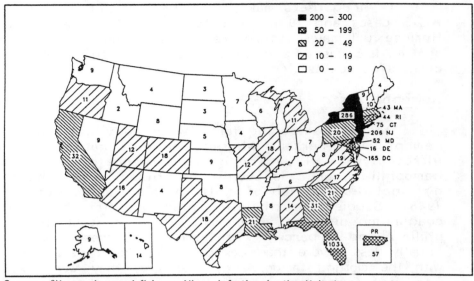

Incidence of AIDS cases in heterosexual adults and adolescents (N = 11,792), by state, per million population, November 2, 1987

Source: "Human Immunodeficiency Virus Infection in the United States," Morbity and Mortality Weekly Report, December 18, 1987.

to which persons at high risk excluded themselves from these groups as well as to the sociodemographic and geographic composition of the groups. When data for a group is adjusted by age, sex, and race, it is not "representative" of the population from which the group is drawn, since representation comes from unbiased sampling. However, adjustment does permit meaningful comparison of data from two different groups. Persons at high risk for infection will undoubtedly be underrepresented among blood donors, military applicants, and Job Corps entrants, three of the five groups investigated, so the detected prevalence among these groups is likely lower than the true prevalence in the segments of the general population from which they come.

Blood Donors

Beginning in 1983, prior to the use of the ELISA (enzyme-linked immunosorbent assay) test (see Chapter II), prospective blood donors were screened for HIV risk factors and those with such factors were requested not to donate blood in an attempt to eliminate donations by those who might have been exposed to the AIDS virus. Because no test existed at that time, there was no way to definitely verify the responses. After 1985, and the advent of ELISA and other screening methods, donated blood and plasma has been screened for the HIV antibody, and blood found to be infected has been discarded.

Among blood donors, a highly selected population, the prevalence for HIV infection is very low, 0.020 percent of 12.6 million American Red Cross donations between April 1985 and May 1987. This data covers 50 percent of all voluntary donations in the U.S. Those who donate for the first time are probably the best source for an estimate of the HIV infection prevalence in the section of the population from which they are drawn, since those who have donated previously and been found to be HIV positive have been identified and eliminated from the donor pool. At this time, there is no national policy for notifying the donor if their blood contains HIV antibody. The Wadley Blood Center in Dallas, Texas notifies all donors of any significant findings regarding the quality of their blood, including the fact that it may test positive for HIV antibody.

HIV antibody prevalence in military applicants (N = 1,253,768), United States, October 1985–September 1987

Percent Antibody Positive

Month

Source: Department of Defense

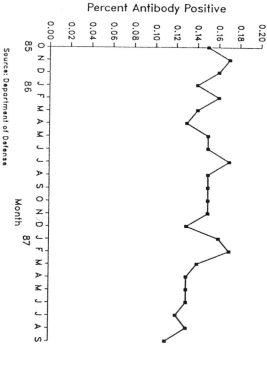

HIV antibody prevalence in military applicants (N = 1,253,768), United States, April 1985–July 1987

Percent Antibody Positive

Month

Source: Department of Defense

HIV antibody prevalence in military applicants (N = 1,253,768) by race or ethnicity, United States, January 1986–September 1987

Percent Antibody Positive

Month

Source: Department of Defense

□ Black (non–Hispanic) : 208,950 tested

● Hispanic : 51,295 tested

○ White (non–Hispanic) : 816,280 tested

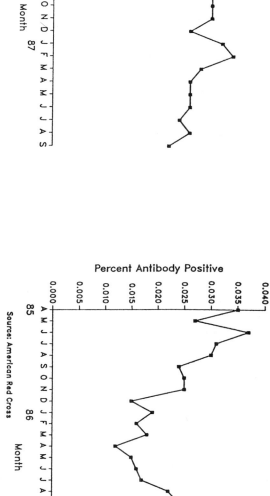

HIV antibody prevalence in blood donors (N = 9,671,411), United States, April 1985–July 1987

Percent Antibody Positive

Month

Source: American Red Cross

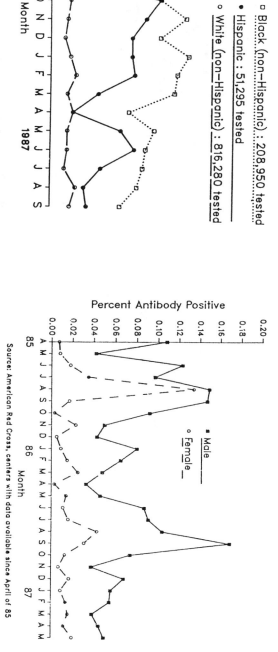

HIV antibody prevalence in first-time blood donors (788,105 males; 726,264 females), by sex, United States, April 1985–May 1987

Percent Antibody Positive

Month

■ Male
○ Female

Source: American Red Cross, centers with data available since April of 85

19

While no statistical or scientific adjustment for age, sex, or race can be made yet, the prevalence rates are considerably higher for men than women, and for blacks and Hispanics than for whites. Despite the fact that blood donors are a highly selected group, of those donors who did test positive, 80 to 90 percent had recognized risk factors for infection.

Military Service Applicants

Since October 1985, all those applying for active duty or reserve military service, the service academies, and the Reserve Officer Training Corps (ROTC) have been screened for HIV infection as part of their medical entrance evaluation. Drug use and homosexual activity are both grounds for exclusion from entry into military service, and applicants are so advised when

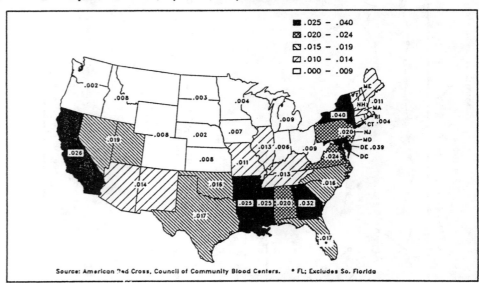

HIV antibody prevalence (percent positive) in blood donors, combined data from adjacent centers, by state, July 1986-June 1987

Source: American Red Cross, Council of Community Blood Centers.   * FL: Excludes So. Florida

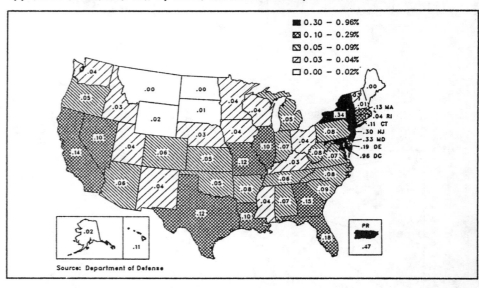

Sex-adjusted HIV antibody prevalence (percent positive) in military applicants (N=1,253,768), by state, October 1985-September 1987

Source: Department of Defense

interviewed by recruiting officials. They are also informed that they will be screened for HIV antibody. Therefore, it would be expected that IV drug users, homosexual and bisexual men, as well as those with coagulant deficiencies, would be underrepresented among military applicants.

Of the almost 1.3 million military applicants evaluated for HIV infection between October 1985 and September 1987, 0.15 percent tested positive. Applicants were mostly male, in a limited age range, and overrepresented by racial and ethnic minorities. When the prevalence rate is corrected to reflect age, sex, and racial and ethnic composition of the U.S. adult population 17-59 years of age, the prevalence barely changed to 0.14 percent.

Job Corps Entrants

The Job Corps is a U.S. Department of Labor program which teaches skills to young people who would otherwise spend most of their adult lives without employment or with under-employment through lack of training. Since March 1987, applicants to residential Job Corps training programs have undergone HIV antibody screening. These are typically disadvantaged youth 16-21 years of age. Those who are part of nonresidential programs are not required to undergo the screening. Testing and counseling are offered, but not required. Neither sexual orientation nor hemophilia is a basis for exclusion, but IV drug use is. Of the initial 25,000 entrants tested, 0.33 percent were HIV positive. This rate is not adjusted for age, sex, or racial or ethnic composition of the group.

Sentinel Hospital Patients

In order to sample a greater cross-section of the population, the CDC initiated a network of sentinel hospitals in September 1986. These 40 hospitals and Health Maintenance Organizations (HMOs) anonymously test the plasma or serum specimens for HIV antibody, of patients of all ages who are being treated for conditions not known to be related to HIV. The CDC hopes this "blind" approach will lessen the chance of a biased selection. The accompanying illustrations show the results from four Midwestern hospitals that participated in the pilot phase of the project. The CDC currently believes this is the closest they can come to objectively sampling trends of the disease in the entire population, since persons in all risk categories can be tested.

The 8,668 test results from the pilot phase showed an overall prevalence of 0.32 percent, with prevalence ranging from 0.09 percent to 0.89 percent. The prevalence rate of military applicants from the same four cities was 0.11 percent.

Nonetheless, even though the samplings at these hospitals were based on the patient's current clinical condition, without regard to risks of HIV infection, hospital patients are not truly representative of their communities, because they are sick. Also, different hospitals serve different segments of the community. Furthermore, many are at high risk, since they have come in for treatment of infectious disease or cancer, or come in through emergency rooms. For example, 6 of 203 critically ill patients (3 percent) in a Baltimore, Maryland emergency room were HIV antibody positive, according to a recent study (Baker, J.L., et al,"Unsuspected human immunodeficiency virus in critically ill emergency patients." Journal of the American Medical Association 1987; 257:-2609-11). Five of these 6 were gunshot or knife wound victims.

Newborn Infants and Women

Virtually all newborns throughout the country are screened for metabolic disorders by filter-paper blood specimens collected from a heel puncture shortly after birth. The Massachusetts Department of Public Health recently developed a method to test these specimen for HIV antibody. Since the tests can detect maternal antibodies which have been passed on to the newborn, this approach finds HIV antibodies among women who have had live births. Numerous studies have found a 30 percent to 50 percent risk that an infected mother will transmit the HIV to her infant. However, an HIV antibody in the newborn does not necessarily mean that the baby has the infection.

HIV antibody prevalence in women of reproductive age, available surveys and studies in settings related to women's health and childbearing, 1984-1987

STATE	CITY	YEAR	TYPE OF CLINIC*	NO. TESTED	PERCENT POSITIVE	REMARKS†	REFERENCE
AL	Montgomery	87	fam plan	694	0.3		B Merrill, AL Hlth Dept, pers com
CA	Alameda Co	85-86	premarital	377	0.5		JAMA 1987;258:474-475
	Los Angeles	87	delivery	500	0.4	WB to be repeated	M Yonekura, Harbor UCLA Med Center, pers com
	Long Beach	86-87	prenatal	227	0.0		H Wallace, Long Beach Hlth Dept, pers com
	Sacramento	87	fam plan	88	0.0		B Hinton, Sacramento Co Hlth Dept, pers com
FL	Jacksonville	86-87	prenatal	299	0.7		A Kaunitz, Univ Hosp, Jacksonville, pers com
IL	Central IL	87	prenatal	97	0.0		N Derrig-Green, priv prac, pers com
	Chicago	86-87	pregnant drug users	150	10.7	40% were IV drug users	I Chasnoff, NW Univ Med Sch, pers com
		86-87	pregnant drug users	102	9.8	primarily IV drug users	S Gall, Univ IL, pers com
MA	Statewide	86-87	newborn (i.e., childbearing women)	30,708	0.2	filter paper test, weighted rate	G Grady, MA Hlth Dept, pers com
MD	Baltimore	85	delivery	678	0.7		T Townsend, J Hopkins Univ, pers com
		86-87	prenatal	115	29.6	only high risk tested	3rd Intl AIDS Conf Abstracts, 1987, MP.85, p24
		86-87	prenatal	88	21.6	only high risk tested	J Johnson, Univ MD, pers com
		87	fam plan	693	0.9		J Modlin, J Hopkins Univ, pers com
MI	Detroit	86-87	pregnant drug users	170	9.4	primarily IV drug users	C Meriwether, Wayne State Univ, pers com
NC	Statewide	87	prenatal	200	0.0		D Jolly, NC Hlth Dept, pers com
	Statewide,	87	fam plan	200	0.0		ibid.
NY	Bronx	87	abortion	351	2.6		Ann Int Med 1987;107:599
NY	Bronx	87	hospital (Beta-HCGS)	820	2.4		E Schoenbaum, Am Publ Hlth Assn meetings, 1987, Late Breaker Session
	Brooklyn	86-87	delivery	602	2.0		S Landesman, JAMA, in press
		86-87	prenatal	255	5.9	Haitian	ibid.
	NYC	86-87	delivery	1,192	2.3		K Krasinski, NYU Sch Med, pers com
PA	Pittsburgh	86-87	fam plan	191	0.0		R Valdessari, Univ Pittsburgh, pers com
PR	San Juan	86-87	delivery	1,036	1.7		C Zorilla, Univ PR Med Sch, pers com
		87	prenatal	2,633	1.7		ibid.
WI	Central WI	86	prenatal	1,000	0.0		P Meier, Marshfield Clinic, pers com

* fam plan = family planning clinic
† WB = Western blot test

Source: "Human Immunodeficiency Virus Infection in the United States," Morbity and Mortality Weekly Report, December 18, 1987.

As of December 1987, Massachusetts is the only state doing the filter-paper blood testing of newborns. Because the testing is blind (no records kept of patient results), the only information is the general location of the hospitals of birth - inner-city, suburban, or rural. In 1986-87, 30,708 tests were performed, with a weighted average prevalence of infection of 0.21 percent for childbearing women statewide. The prevalence varied from 0.80 percent at inner-city hospitals to 0.09 percent at suburban and rural hospitals. This compares to the crude prevalence rate of 0.13 percent for female military applicants from Massachusetts.

The CDC bases its prevalence reporting on 27 studies of women in health and childbearing settings. These studies conducted in 19 cities in 12 states were targeted on inner-city areas where considerable levels of infection were anticipated because of likely higher rate of existing AIDS cases and more frequent IV drug use. With the exception of women expected to be at high risk for HIV infection because of drug use, the findings ranged from a fraction of 1 percent in most areas to as high as 2.6 percent in New York City and Puerto Rico. Some extreme rates as high as 30 percent have been found among groups of pregnant drug users. (See Chapter VI, for a more detailed study of children and AIDS)

CHAPTER IV

GEOGRAPHY, DEMOGRAPHY AND PREVALENCE

While all Americans could possibly become infected with the AIDS virus under the proper condition, where a person lives and who a person is plays an enormous role in the likelihood of getting AIDS. The consequences of behavior can vary dramatically depending upon geography and demography.

GEOGRAPHY AND BEHAVIOR

AIDS cases and HIV antibody prevalence vary significantly by geographic area. New York, with 693 AIDS cases per 1 million population, has the highest rate in the nation. On the other hand, North and South Dakota, with 9 and 7, cases per million, respectively, have not suffered nearly the impact that other, more populated states have had.

While homosexual men and intravenous drug users are most likely to have AIDS, geography plays an important role as well. As Patricia Gadsby, in "Mapping The Epidemic: Geography as Destiny," (Discover, Vol. 8, No. 4, April 1988), points out, someone is 15 times more likely to become infected with AIDS in the Manhattan borough of New York City than in Manhattan, Kansas.

New York State and California are the two states hardest hit initially by the epidemic. The CDC reports that in 1982, 71 percent of all AIDS cases were concentrated in these two states. By early 1988, however, other areas of the country were being hit to the point that New York and California represented only 48 percent of the cases.

Although these two states still have high rate of AIDS, the victims in each state differ. Homosexual and bisexual men account for the overwhelming majority of AIDS cases in California. They tend to be educated, middle-class, white, relatively affluent men. On the other hand, the people in New York, and portions of New Jersey, most subject to AIDS infection are poor, inner-city minorities who are IV drug abusers or sexual partners or children of women who are IV drug abusers. In 1987, AIDS-related deaths among IV drug users in New York City passed that of homosexual men. New York City health officials fear that half of that city's IV drug users are infected with the virus, compared with 5 percent of users in most U.S. cities.

Dr. Ernest Drucker, a New York epidemiologist and head of the community health and drug addiction programs at Montefiore Medical Center in the Bronx, feels that public health officials, focusing on who gets AIDS with respect to risky behavior, have overlooked geography as a factor in targeting preventive measures. It may not be so much what you do, as where you do it. If there is no virus around, Dr. Drucker points out, you won't get AIDS. If the AIDS virus is prevalent in an area, the risk of infection is high.

Many men in poor minority areas of New York are intravenous drug users and engage in heterosexual activity. Because they tend to stay in their own neighborhoods, the women in the neighborhoods are the ones with whom they have sex. Needless to say, the infection rate could skyrocket. Dr. Drucker reports that in some areas of New York, one in five men tested positive for infection. Their sexual partners are at very, very high risk. Unfortunately, the transmission of the infection does not stop there, since the newborn babies of these women are also at high risk.

Race and Ethnicity

Blacks and Hispanics (who can be of any color) are disproportionately represented among AIDS victims. While they are 12 and 7 percent of the U.S. population, respectively, they constitute 24 percent and 14 percent of the cases of AIDS, according to Dr. Donald

Incidence of AIDS cases (N=44,745), by state, per million population, November 2, 1987

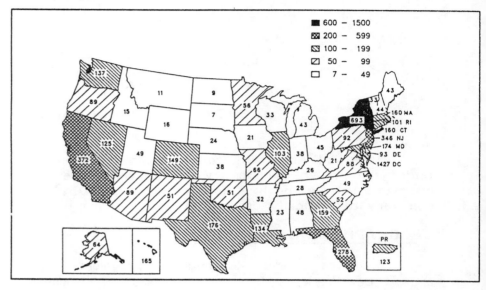

HIV antibody prevalence (percent positive), averaged from multiple studies, in homosexual men (A), IV drug users (B), and hemophiliacs (C), selected areas, United States

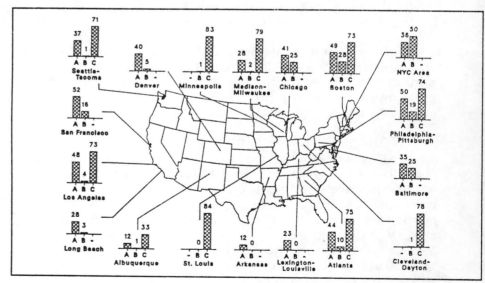

Source: "Human Immunodeficiency Virus Infection in the United States," Morbity and Mortality Weekly Report, December 18, 1987.

AIDS CASES BY STATE OF RESIDENCE AND DATE OF REPORT TO CDC

STATE OF RESIDENCE	Year Ending MAY 23, 1987		Year Ending MAY 23, 1988		CUMULATIVE TOTAL SINCE JUNE 1981					
					Adult/Adolescent		Children		Total	
	Number	Percent	Number	Percent	Number	Percent	Number	Percent	Number	Percent
New York	3743	(24.5)	5479	(20.7)	15855	(25.7)	308	(31.1)	16163	(25.8)
California	3301	(21.6)	5513	(20.8)	13428	(21.7)	74	(7.5)	13502	(21.5)
Florida	1140	(7.5)	1881	(7.1)	4340	(7.0)	117	(11.8)	4457	(7.1)
Texas	1192	(7.8)	1818	(6.9)	4083	(6.6)	38	(3.8)	4121	(6.6)
New Jersey	885	(5.8)	1967	(7.4)	3989	(6.5)	129	(13.0)	4118	(6.6)
Illinois	459	(3.0)	798	(3.0)	1722	(2.8)	24	(2.4)	1746	(2.8)
Pennsylvania	365	(2.4)	800	(3.0)	1625	(2.6)	22	(2.2)	1647	(2.6)
Georgia	386	(2.5)	570	(2.1)	1308	(2.1)	20	(2.0)	1328	(2.1)
Massachusetts	341	(2.2)	543	(2.0)	1280	(2.1)	22	(2.2)	1302	(2.1)
District of Columbia	306	(2.0)	507	(1.9)	1177	(1.9)	12	(1.2)	1189	(1.9)
Maryland	274	(1.8)	482	(1.8)	1046	(1.7)	21	(2.1)	1067	(1.7)
Puerto Rico	118	(0.8)	649	(2.4)	969	(1.6)	37	(3.7)	1006	(1.6)
Washington	238	(1.6)	387	(1.5)	834	(1.4)	4	(0.4)	838	(1.3)
Louisiana	197	(1.3)	401	(1.5)	821	(1.3)	11	(1.1)	832	(1.3)
Ohio	216	(1.4)	432	(1.6)	793	(1.3)	14	(1.4)	807	(1.3)
Connecticut	177	(1.2)	329	(1.2)	726	(1.2)	28	(2.8)	754	(1.2)
Virginia	178	(1.2)	300	(1.1)	708	(1.1)	15	(1.5)	723	(1.2)
Colorado	185	(1.2)	294	(1.1)	665	(1.1)	5	(0.5)	670	(1.1)
Michigan	180	(1.2)	302	(1.1)	633	(1.0)	10	(1.0)	643	(1.0)
Missouri	130	(0.9)	318	(1.2)	546	(0.9)	7	(0.7)	553	(0.9)
Arizona	66	(0.4)	326	(1.2)	504	(0.8)	3	(0.3)	507	(0.8)
North Carolina	99	(0.6)	275	(1.0)	485	(0.8)	9	(0.9)	494	(0.8)
Oregon	78	(0.5)	199	(0.8)	354	(0.6)	2	(0.2)	356	(0.6)
Minnesota	105	(0.7)	134	(0.5)	337	(0.5)	2	(0.2)	339	(0.5)
Tennessee	56	(0.4)	220	(0.8)	318	(0.5)	5	(0.5)	323	(0.5)
Indiana	76	(0.5)	161	(0.6)	318	(0.5)	3	(0.3)	321	(0.5)
Alabama	71	(0.5)	182	(0.7)	295	(0.5)	10	(1.0)	305	(0.5)
South Carolina	66	(0.4)	108	(0.4)	242	(0.4)	5	(0.5)	247	(0.4)
Oklahoma	62	(0.4)	112	(0.4)	218	(0.4)	6	(0.6)	224	(0.4)
Hawaii	84	(0.5)	81	(0.3)	221	(0.4)	1	(0.1)	222	(0.4)
Wisconsin	63	(0.4)	103	(0.4)	215	(0.3)	1	(0.1)	216	(0.3)
Nevada	53	(0.3)	114	(0.4)	202	(0.3)	2	(0.2)	204	(0.3)
Kentucky	34	(0.2)	68	(0.3)	147	(0.2)			147	(0.2)
Mississippi	32	(0.2)	95	(0.4)	144	(0.2)			144	(0.2)
Rhode Island	46	(0.3)	67	(0.3)	141	(0.2)	3	(0.3)	144	(0.2)
Kansas	44	(0.3)	67	(0.3)	140	(0.2)	2	(0.2)	142	(0.2)
Arkansas	32	(0.2)	69	(0.3)	127	(0.2)			127	(0.2)
Utah	26	(0.2)	63	(0.2)	121	(0.2)	3	(0.3)	124	(0.2)
New Mexico	32	(0.2)	52	(0.2)	107	(0.2)	1	(0.1)	108	(0.2)
Delaware	23	(0.2)	45	(0.2)	94	(0.2)	2	(0.2)	96	(0.2)
Iowa	23	(0.2)	29	(0.1)	73	(0.1)	2	(0.2)	75	(0.1)
Maine	23	(0.2)	32	(0.1)	73	(0.1)	2	(0.2)	75	(0.1)
New Hampshire	17	(0.1)	38	(0.1)	65	(0.1)	3	(0.3)	68	(0.1)
Nebraska	18	(0.1)	31	(0.1)	62	(0.1)			62	(0.1)
West Virginia	14	(0.1)	18	(0.1)	45	(0.1)	2	(0.2)	47	(0.1)
Alaska	10	(0.1)	18	(0.1)	45	(0.1)			45	(0.1)
Vermont	8	(0.1)	15	(0.1)	29	(0.0)			29	(0.0)
Montana	4	(0.0)	12	(0.0)	20	(0.0)			20	(0.0)
Idaho	5	(0.0)	10	(0.0)	17	(0.0)	2	(0.2)	19	(0.0)
Virgin Islands	2	(0.0)	9	(0.0)	15	(0.0)	1	(0.1)	16	(0.0)
Wyoming	4	(0.0)	2	(0.0)	9	(0.0)			9	(0.0)
South Dakota	2	(0.0)	4	(0.0)	8	(0.0)			8	(0.0)
North Dakota	2	(0.0)			6	(0.0)			6	(0.0)
Guam			3	(0.0)	4	(0.0)			4	(0.0)
Trust Territory					1	(0.0)			1	(0.0)
TOTAL	15291	(100.0)	26532	(100.0)	61750	(100.0)	990	(100.0)	62740	(100.0)

Source: "AIDS Weekly Surveillance Report,"
Centers for Disease Control, May 23, 1988

AIDS CASES BY TRANSMISSION CATEGORIES AND DATE OF REPORT TO CDC, TWELVE-MONTH TOTALS

TRANSMISSION CATEGORIES [1]	Year Ending MAY 23, 1987		Year Ending MAY 23, 1988		CUMULATIVE CASES AND DEATHS SINCE JUNE 1981			
ADULTS/ADOLESCENTS	Number	(%)	Number	(%)	Number	(%)	Deaths	(% Cases)
Homosexual/Bisexual Male	9985	(66.3)	15481	(59.4)	39001	(63.2)	21661	(62.6)
Intravenous (IV) Drug Abuser	2406	(16.0)	5485	(21.0)	11524	(18.7)	6396	(18.5)
Homosexual Male and IV Drug Abuser	1087	(7.2)	1825	(7.0)	4568	(7.4)	2731	(7.9)
Hemophilia/Coagulation Disorder	175	(1.2)	261	(1.0)	606	(1.0)	357	(1.0)
Heterosexual Cases [2]	604	(4.0)	1112	(4.3)	2535	(4.1)	1358	(3.9)
Transfusion, Blood/Components	395	(2.6)	790	(3.0)	1527	(2.5)	1032	(3.0)
Undetermined [3]	412	(2.7)	1111	(4.3)	1989	(3.2)	1073	(3.1)
SUBTOTAL	15064	(100.0)	26065	(100.0)	61750	(100.0)	34608	(100.0)
CHILDREN [4]								
Hemophilia/Coagulation Disorder	14	(6.2)	29	(6.2)	56	(5.7)	34	(5.9)
Parent with/at risk of AIDS [5]	186	(81.9)	349	(74.7)	762	(77.0)	441	(76.0)
Transfusion, Blood/Components	21	(9.3)	66	(14.1)	134	(13.5)	82	(14.1)
Undetermined [3]	6	(2.6)	23	(4.9)	38	(3.8)	23	(4.0)
SUBTOTAL	227	(100.0)	467	(100.0)	990	(100.0)	580	(100.0)
TOTAL	15291		26532		62740		35188	

[1] Cases with more than one risk factor other than the combinations listed in the tables or footnotes are tabulated only in the category listed first.

[2] IncTudes 1518 persons (327 men, 1191 women) who have had heterosexual contact with a person with AIDS or at risk for AIDS and 1017 persons (793 men, 224 women) without other identified risks who were born in countries in which heterosexual transmission is believed to play a major role although precise means of transmission have not yet been fully defined.

[3] Includes patients on whom risk information is incomplete (due to death, refusal to be interviewed or loss to

Source: "AIDS Weekly Surveillance Report,"
Centers for Disease Control, May 23, 1988

Hopkins in "AIDS in Minority Populations in the United States" (Public Health Reports, November-December 1987, Vol. 102, No.6, pp. 677-681. May 1988 statistics show blacks with 26 percent of all reported cases, while the Hispanic proportion remained unchanged). To date, the relative risk to other minorities, Native Americans, Asians, and Pacific Islanders has been small. This does not mean that they are not at risk, nor that they do not need to take the necessary precautions everyone should take.

Of the AIDS cases reported in the U.S. as of May 23, 1988, 36,823 were white, 16,282 were black, and 9,050 were Hispanic. Although a majority were whites (59 percent), the proportions among blacks and Hispanics were twice their proportion of the population. AIDS in children is tragic. Minority children (those under age 13) are hit especially hard with AIDS infection since it often is in addition to the problems of poverty and broken homes which many of them face. Among children with AIDS, 53 percent are black, 22 percent are Hispanic, and 24 percent are white - three-quarters of all children with AIDS are minorities. Black women represent 52 percent of all cases among women, and Hispanic women are 19 percent.

Although blacks become infected with HIV the same ways other AIDS victims do, sexually, perinatally (time closely surrounding time of birth), or parenterally (through IV drug abuse or transfusion), there are significant differences in the proportion of those infected by the different methods of transmission. Twelve percent of white men who have AIDS are IV drug users or had sex partners who were IV drug users; 40 percent of black and Hispanic men fall in that category. Nearly half of all white women with AIDS (47.8 percent) were either IV drug users or had sex partners who were; 70 percent of all black women with AIDS and 83 percent of all Hispanic women with AIDS had these characteristics.

Among children with AIDS, less than one-third of white victims (30.8 percent) were born to mothers who also had AIDS or whose sex partner had AIDS. On the other hand, 61 percent of black and 76 percent of Hispanic children were infected by this method of transmission.

AIDS CASES BY DATE OF DIAGNOSIS AND STANDARD METROPOLITAN STATISTICAL AREA (SMSA) OF RESIDENCE[6]

SMSA OF RESIDENCE	POPULATION[7]	BEFORE 1985	1985	1986	1987	1988[8]	CUMULATIVE TOTAL
New York, NY	9.12	3295	2626	3544	3959	1069	14493
San Francisco, CA	3.25	1089	972	1425	1555	446	5487
Los Angeles, CA	7.48	810	882	1355	1580	263	4890
Houston, TX	2.91	293	340	618	690	73	2014
Washington, DC	3.06	221	341	455	686	192	1895
Newark, NJ	1.97	269	270	422	689	125	1775
Miami, FL	1.63	378	295	409	441	61	1584
Chicago, IL	7.10	200	233	401	591	148	1573
Philadelphia, PA	4.72	175	210	339	474	95	1293
Dallas, TX	2.97	117	178	336	551	60	1242
Atlanta, GA	2.03	112	168	273	350	81	984
Boston, MA	2.76	139	153	216	342	84	934
San Diego, CA	1.86	78	118	218	317	97	828
Ft Lauderdale, FL	1.02	97	131	209	292	68	797
Jersey City, NJ	0.56	115	144	208	251	38	756
Nassau-Suffolk, NY	2.61	123	124	207	215	54	723
Seattle, WA	1.61	66	94	180	238	61	639
New Orleans, LA	1.19	70	97	151	216	38	572
Denver,CO	1.62	63	85	140	204	74	566
Baltimore, MD	2.17	59	81	140	222	51	553
REST OF U.S.	168.48	2211	2883	4900	7458	1690	19142
TOTAL	230.11	9980	10425	16146	21321	4868	62740

[7] Population of SMSA's in millions as reported in the 1980 CENSUS.

[8] Cases diagnosed in this calendar year and reported to CDC as of date of this summary.

Source: "AIDS Weekly Surveillance Report,"
Centers for Disease Control, May 23, 1988

Drug abuse, which took its toll in minority communities long before the onset of the AIDS epidemic, has now taken on an even more menacing role. Minority babies, who are frequently born without the benefit of prenatal care and are thus subject to a slower, shakier start than other babies, now face the even dimmer prospect of being born to die.

The concentration of minorities with AIDS is consistent with the geography of AIDS victims who are primarily drug abusers. Virtually two-thirds of black (58 percent) and Hispanic (61 percent) adults with AIDS reside in New York, New Jersey, or Florida. However, even among drug abusers in New York City, there are important racial, cultural, and economic differences. The CDC reports ("Prevalence of and risk factors associated with HTLV III/LAV antibodies among intravenous drug abusers in methadone program in New York City," presented at the International Conference on AIDS, Paris, France, June 1986 and reported in Morbity and Mortality Weekly Reports, October 26, 1986) that among IV drug abusers in New York City, the prevalence of HIV antibody was only 14 percent among white patients, but 42 percent for black and Hispanic patients. A higher proportion of white patients (18 percent) than black or Hispanic patients (8 percent) reported using new needles at least half the time when they injected drugs. Blacks and Hispanics were less educated than their white counterparts and more likely to be receiving public assistance. Because of the high incidence of perinatally-transmitted AIDS due to IV drug use, it is not surprising that 73 percent of black children and 63 percent of the Hispanic children with AIDS also lived in the three states mentioned as well.

TRANSMISSION CATEGORIES BY RACIAL/ETHNIC GROUP	WHITE, NOT HISPANIC		BLACK, NOT HISPANIC		HISPANIC		OTHER[8]/ UNKNOWN		TOTAL	
ADULTS/ADOLESCENTS	Cumulative Number	(%)	Cumulative Number	(%)	Cumulative Number	(%)	Cumulative Number	(%)	Cumulative Number	(%)
Homosexual/Bisexual Male	28710	(78)	6010	(38)	3891	(44)	390	(68)	39001	(63)
Intravenous (IV) Drug Abuser	2229	(6)	5846	(37)	3392	(38)	57	(10)	11524	(19)
Homosexual Male and IV Drug Abuser	2796	(8)	1111	(7)	638	(7)	23	(4)	4568	(7)
Hemophilia/Coagulation Disorder	513	(1)	41	(0)	40	(0)	12	(2)	606	(1)
Heterosexual Cases[3]	458	(1)	1723	(11)	342	(4)	12	(2)	2535	(4)
Transfusion, Blood/Components	1136	(3)	234	(1)	119	(1)	38	(7)	1527	(2)
Undetermined[4]	747	(2)	793	(5)	406	(5)	43	(7)	1989	(3)
SUBTOTAL [% of all cases]	36589	[59]	15758	[26]	8828	[14]	575	[1]	61750	[100]
CHILDREN[5]										
Hemophilia/Coagulation Disorder	41	(18)	6	(1)	7	(3)	2	(20)	56	(6)
Parent with/at risk of AIDS[6]	111	(47)	464	(89)	180	(81)	7	(70)	762	(77)
Transfusion, Blood/Components	75	(32)	31	(6)	27	(12)	1	(10)	134	(14)
Undetermined[4]	7	(3)	23	(4)	8	(4)			38	(4)
SUBTOTAL [% of all cases]	234	[24]	524	[53]	222	[22]	10	[1]	990	[100]
TOTAL [% of all cases]	36823	[59]	16282	[26]	9050	[14]	585	[1]	62740[7]	[100]

[8] Includes patients whose race/ethnicity is Asian/Pacific Islander (367 persons) and American Indian/Alaskan Native (64 persons).

AGE AT DIAGNOSIS BY RACIAL/ETHNIC GROUP	WHITE, NOT HISPANIC		BLACK, NOT HISPANIC		HISPANIC		OTHER[5]/ UNKNOWN		TOTAL	
AGE GROUP	Cumulative Number	(%)	Cumulative Number	(%)	Cumulative Number	(%)	Cumulative Number	(%)	Cumulative Number	(%)
Under 5	159	(0)	469	(3)	197	(2)	8	(1)	833	(1)
5 - 12	75	(0)	55	(0)	25	(0)	2	(0)	157	(0)
13 - 19	125	(0)	89	(1)	46	(1)	5	(1)	265	(0)
20 - 29	6984	(19)	3787	(23)	2102	(23)	104	(18)	12977	(21)
30 - 39	16722	(45)	7851	(48)	4250	(47)	254	(43)	29077	(46)
40 - 49	8309	(23)	2820	(17)	1754	(19)	142	(24)	13025	(21)
Over 49	4449	(12)	1211	(7)	676	(7)	70	(12)	6406	(10)
TOTAL [% OF ALL CASES]	36823	[59]	16282	[26]	9050	[14]	585	[1]	62740	[100]

[5] Includes patients whose race/ethnicity is Asian/Pacific Islander (367 persons) and American Indian/Alaskan Native (64 persons).

Source: "AIDS Weekly Surveillance Report," Centers for Disease Control, May 23, 1988

A very real threat for all communities, but particularly minority communities, is from infected, asymptomatic, infectious persons who have sexual relations with others or who share IV drug needles with others. Minorities showed higher prevalence rates of HIV-positivity among civilian applicants for military services and blood donors than whites. Dr. James Curran, Director of the AIDS Project in the Center for Infectious Diseases at CDC, has calculated that if the estimated 1.5 million Americans believed to be infected with the AIDS virus are distributed similarly to the 60,000 already diagnosed so far, the results would be - 0.5 percent of the white U.S. population are infected with HIV, while about 1.5 percent of the blacks and Hispanic populations are infected. Some studies in predominantly black and Hispanic neighborhoods have found proportions even higher. AIDS is a problem of the heterosexual black and Hispanic communities. Almost half of the blacks and Hispanics with AIDS are heterosexual, compared with less than 15 percent of whites with AIDS.

Minority Distinctions

Of the Hispanics with AIDS who live in the northeastern U.S., 80-90 percent were born in Puerto Rico. In Florida, one-third of the blacks with AIDS were born in Haiti. Problems with reaching and educating certain blacks and Hispanics include language barriers and differences in the media channels these groups patronize. Many in these groups are also painfully aware of their minority status in this country and may fear that efforts to reach those with AIDS are just another excuse for discrimination. A number of minorities, especially first-generation immigrants, have a suspicion of things connected with the government, as most educational and fact-finding contacts would be.

CHAPTER V

WOMEN, HETEROSEXUALS, AND AIDS

As noted in the opening chapters, AIDS was initially known as the "gay disease" because homosexuals were the first in this country to be diagnosed as being infected. Until scientists discovered that a virus caused AIDS and that it could be transmitted through "bodily fluids", such as semen and blood, those who were not "gay," namely women and heterosexuals believed they had little to fear. The rise in reported cases among women and heterosexuals, however, has made everyone realize that few are untouched by this virus, if proper precautions are not taken and education is not available.

WOMEN

In late 1986, when Dr. Mary Guinan and Ann Hardy of the Centers for Disease Control began their analysis, only 1,189 cases of AIDS had been reported in women since 1981, less than 7 percent of all cases at that time. By May 1988, over 4,800 women had become infected with AIDS, although this still represented only about 8 percent of adults with AIDS. Occurrences of AIDS and HIV infection in women is particularly important because they are the major source of infections in infants. This, coupled with the fact that heterosexual transmission is the second most common method of transmission of AIDS to women, behind intravenous drug use, provides important information to predict the trends for cases among children and may help monitor heterosexual transmission of the infection.

Characteristics

Between 1982 and 1986, the period of this study, the proportion of women with AIDS had not changed dramatically. Women with AIDS tended to be considerably younger than non-homosexual/bisexual men with AIDS. Almost one-third were in the 20- to 29-year age group, compared with one-fifth of the men. The overwhelming majority of women with AIDS were in child-bearing years - 79 percent were between 13 and 39. Over half of the women were black, and another 20 percent were Hispanic.

Geography

By 1986, 43 states, Puerto Rico, and the District of Columbia, had reported cases of AIDS in women. Geographically, the distribution of women with AIDS was similar to that of men. New York had the highest number of cases for both sexes (7,727 men and 855 women). California had the second highest number of men (6,068), but the fourth largest number of women (106). The highest proportion of women with AIDS were found in New Jersey and Connecticut (16 percent), Puerto Rico (12 percent), Florida and Rhode Island (12 percent), and New York (10 percent).

Transmission

Over half of the women with AIDS (52 percent) were infected through intravenous drug use, while 21 percent were infected through heterosexual contact with a person who was at risk for AIDS. Only 1 percent of non-homosexual/bisexual men with AIDS were known to have been infected through heterosexual contact. Of those adults with AIDS whose only risk factor was heterosexual contact, 84 percent were women.

Of the women who became infected due to heterosexual contact, 67 percent had had contact with an intravenous drug user; 16 percent had had contact with bisexual men, 1 percent with men who were hemophiliacs; and 16 percent with men with other or unreported risk factors. If homosexual/-bisexual men were not counted, the overall ratio of men with AIDS to women with AIDS was 3:1. The ratio was far higher for those with hemophilia/-coagulation disorders, which is not surprising since hemophilia strikes far more men than women.

—Men and Women With Adult AIDS, 1981 Through 1986,* Excluding Homosexual and Bisexual Men, by Age Group, Race, and Disease

	No. (%) of Cases	
	Men	Women
Age, y		
13-19	39 (1)	21 (1)
20-29	1031 (20)	588 (32)†
30-39	2681 (50)	821 (45)
40-49	973 (18)	197 (11)‡
>49	634 (12)	192 (11)
Race		
White	1342 (25)	502 (28)
Black	2622 (49)	930 (51)
Hispanic	1343 (25)	365 (20)
Other	30 (1)	14 (1)
Unreported	21 (<1)	8 (<1)
Diseases		
Kaposi's sarcoma	201 (4)	48 (3)
Pneumocystis carinii pneumonia	3558 (66)	1203 (66)
Kaposi's sarcoma and *P carinii* pneumonia	49 (1)	10 (<1)
Other	1550 (29)	558 (31)

*Cases reported through Nov 7, 1986.
†Men vs women, P<.001.
‡Men vs women, P<.01.

Source: "Epidemiology of AIDS in Women in the United States," *Journal of the American Medical Association*, April 17, 1987

—Temporal Trends in AIDS, 1982 Through 1986*

Transmission Category	% of Cases				
	1982	1983	1984	1985	1986*
Homosexual/bisexual					
Men	77	77	79	79	79
Women	0	0	0	0	0
Intravenous drug user					
Men	15	16	14	15	14
Women	47	59	56	52	48
Hemophilia/coagulation disorder					
Men	0.9	0.5	0.8	1	1
Women	0	0	1	0.2	0.4
Heterosexual contact*					
Men	0.2	0.1	0.3	0.3	0.4
Women	14	14	17	20	26
Born in country with heterosexual transmission					
Men	5	4	2	1	1
Women	18	8	6	5	5
Transfusion					
Men	0.3	0.7	0.8	1.3	1.5
Women	8	7	8	11	10
Undetermined					
Men	2	3	2	2	3
Women	14	12	12	11	10

*With person at risk for AIDS.
*Cases reported as of Nov 7, 1986. Some of these cases are still being investigated and may be reclassified.

Mothers and Children

With the exception of one risk group, the increase in the number of women with AIDS was comparable to the increase in child patients whose mothers were members of these risk groups. The one exception was the trend among women and children with AIDS whose mothers were born in a country where heterosexual transmission was the common method of transmission, in which case, the rate of AIDS cases in the children, was greater than that of the mothers.

Researchers' Observations

Since heterosexual contact is the only transmission category where women outnumber men, a heterosexual woman is at greater risk for becoming infected with AIDS through sexual intercourse than a heterosexual man. There are probably two reasons for the larger number of heterosexually-acquired AIDS cases among women – a greater proportion of men are infected, therefore, a woman is more likely to encounter an infected man; and the virus may be transmitted more efficiently from man to woman than from woman to man.

Anal intercourse has played a large role in the high risk for AIDS and HIV antibody among homosexual men, but it does not seem to be a major factor among heterosexual women. While the study mentioned above did not determine the risk, other studies have shown a low incidence of anal intercourse among infected women, which suggests that women contract AIDS through other types of sexual contact.

A few cases of women contracting AIDS through artificial insemination into the uterus with a catheter of infected semen have been recorded. This confirms that vaginal-penile intercourse presumably can be a method of transmission. The researchers of this study did not determine if the risk of infection was greater if the virus entered through the anus or the vagina, however, but other authorities believe that because of the thin lining of the rectum, and the proximity of blood vessels, the rectum is more susceptible to rupture and infection. Direct contact between the virus and blood occurs when skin and mucous membranes are not intact, which is most often the case in anal intercourse. However, Dr. Guinan and Ms. Hardy observe, if HIV can pass through membranes which are intact, (which research has shown), the risk of transmission through the vagina or the rectum may be no different.

Ten percent of women, versus 3 percent of men,

—Adult Men and Women With AIDS, Excluding Homosexual and Bisexual Men, by Sex and Transmission Category, 1981 Through 1986*

	No. (%) of Cases		
Risk Group	Men	Women	M-F Ratio
Intravenous drug use	3654 (68)	940 (52)	4:1
Hemophilia/coagulation disorder	232 (4)	7 (<1)	33:1
Heterosexual contact†	75 (1)	381 (21)‡	0.2:1
Born in country with heterosexual transmission	451 (8)	110 (6)	4:1
Transfusions	309 (6)	180 (10)	2:1
Undetermined	637 (12)	201 (11)	3:1
Total	5358	1819	3:1

*Cases reported as of Nov 7, 1986.
†Heterosexual contact with a person at risk for AIDS.
‡Men vs women, P<.0001.

—Adult Men and Women With AIDS in the United States, 1981 Through 1986

	Women	Men	Total	% Female of Total
1981*	6	196	202	3.0
1982	51	687	738	6.9
1983	162	2213	2375	6.8
1984	302	4384	4686	6.4
1985	569	8062	8631	6.6
1986†	729	9775	10 504	6.9

*Reporting initiated in late spring of 1981.
†Cases reported through Nov 7, 1986.

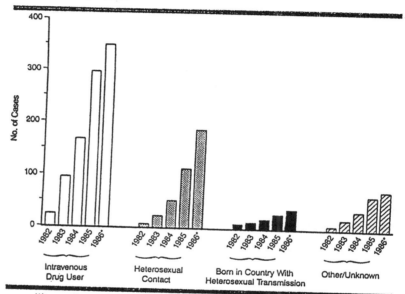

—Women with acquired immunodeficiency syndrome, by risk group, 1982 through 1986. Asterisk indicates that 1986 data are through Nov 7, 1986.

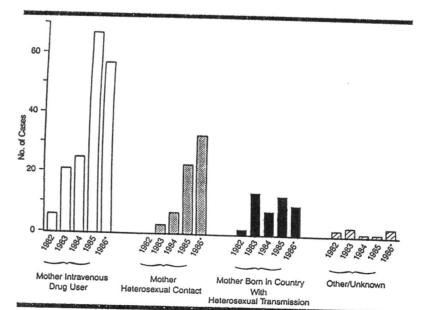

—Children with acquired immunodeficiency syndrome, by maternal risk group, 1982 through 1986. Asterisk indicates that 1986 data are through Nov 7, 1986.

Source: "Epidemiology of AIDS in Women in the United States," Journal of the American Medical Association, April 17, 1987

with AIDS have no identified risk. Perhaps one reason is the that some women do not know that a person is in a high-risk group, i.e. intravenous drug user or bisexual. Most men do not introduce themselves at a party as being either of these. Women who engage in casual sex, especially those residing in areas such as New York City and San Francisco, should realize they are at high risk.

If present trends continue, the number of infants born with AIDS to mothers who are at an undetermined risk or are at risk through heterosexual contact with an infected person will increase. The primary problem is that these women may be unaware of their risk and, therefore, not receive counseling or testing before becoming pregnant. Preventing HIV infection in women is absolutely necessary to prevent the majority of AIDS cases in children whose mothers are in these categories. Some areas hardest hit have already begun counseling women who are IV drug users.

Because it is difficult to identify and target women who are at higher risks, all women need to be aware of the risks of sexually-acquired AIDS and encouraged to engage in behavior which reduces their risks, such as celibacy and monogamy. Women who are sexually active with more than one partner and those whose partners are HIV-infected or at high risk should insist that their partners always use condoms.

HETEROSEXUAL RISK

Because AIDS is incurable, the only method to control the disease is to control the spread of infection through prevention. Blood products must be made safe to prevent infection through infusion or inoculation. To prevent the perinatal spread of infection in newborns, mothers must be tested before becoming pregnant and advised against having children, or if already pregnant, some health personnel believe, to consider abortion. The most common means of spreading the HIV infection is through sexual contact. Responsible health personnel advise limiting sexual partners, using condoms, and avoiding high-risk activities such as anal intercourse. Some authorities advice the more difficult to follow restriction of avoiding sex with anyone who has not been tested for HIV antibody and shown to be uninfected. Drs. Norman Hearst and Stephen B. Hulley, two eminent San Francisco physicians actively involved in the epidemiology of AIDS, concluded in "Preventing the Heterosexual Spread of AIDS: Are We Giving Our Patients the Best Advice?" (Journal of the American Medical Association, April 19, 1988, Vol. 259, No.16, pp. 2428-2432) that the most important advice physicians can give their patients is to avoid sexual contact with a person who may be at high risk.

Risk Estimates

The accompanying table presents estimates of the risk of HIV infection to an uninfected person based on one heterosexual encounter and on five years of frequent heterosexual encounters with different types of partners. The risk involved is based on three factors: 1) the likelihood that the partner has the virus; 2) the likelihood of infection from a single sexual encounter with an infected person; and 3) the reduction of risks with use of condoms and spermicides (chemicals which kill active sperm).

The risks vary dramatically. The lowest risk is 1 in 5 billion for a single sexual encounter using a condom with person at low risk who has tested seronegative for the HIV antibody. The highest risk is 2 in 3 for 500 sexual encounters without using a condom with a partner known to be infected. The choice of 500 sexual encounters was based on the median time between HIV in-

Risk Category of Partner	Assumptions			Estimated Risk of Infection	
	Prevalence of HIV Infection	Infectivity†	Condom/Spermicide Failure Rate	1 Sexual Encounter‡	500 Sexual Encounters§
HIV serostatus unknown					
Not in any high-risk group					
Using condoms	0.0001	0.002	0.1	1 in 50 000 000	1 in 110 000
Not using condoms	0.0001	0.002	...	1 in 5 000 000	1 in 16 000
High-risk groups‖					
Using condoms	0.05 to 0.5	0.002	0.1	1 in 100 000 to 1 in 10 000	1 in 210 to 1 in 21
Not using condoms	0.05 to 0.5	0.002	...	1 in 10 000 to 1 in 1000	1 in 32 to 1 in 3
HIV seronegative					
No history of high-risk behavior¶					
Using condoms	0.000001	0.002	0.1	1 in 5 000 000 000	1 in 11 000 000
Not using condoms	0.000001	0.002	...	1 in 500 000 000	1 in 1 600 000
Continuing high-risk behavior¶					
Using condoms	0.01	0.002	0.1	1 in 500 000	1 in 1100
Not using condoms	0.01	0.002	...	1 in 50 000	1 in 160
HIV seropositive					
Using condoms	1.0	0.002	0.1	1 in 5000	1 in 11
Not using condoms	1.0	0.002	...	1 in 500	2 in 3

*HIV indicates human immunodeficiency virus.

†The value 0.002 represents an upper limit on the probability that an infected male will transmit HIV to an uninfected female during one episode of penile-vaginal intercourse with ejaculation. Female-to-male infectivity may be lower, and infectivity for anal intercourse or intercourse when genital ulcers are present may be higher. The value is a group mean and may vary among individuals.

‡The risk of infection for one encounter is the product of the values in columns 2 through 4 of the Table ("Assumptions").

§The risk of infection for 500 encounters is column $2 \times [1 - (1 - \text{column } 3 \times \text{column } 4)^{500}]$.

‖High-risk groups with prevalences of HIV infection at the higher end of the range given include homosexual or bisexual men and intravenous drug users from major metropolitan areas, and hemophiliacs. Groups with prevalences at the lower end of the range include homosexual or bisexual men and intravenous drug users from other parts of the country, female prostitutes, heterosexuals from countries where heterosexual spread of HIV is common (including Haiti and central Africa), and recipients of multiple blood transfusions between 1983 and 1985 from areas with a high prevalence of HIV infection.

¶High-risk behavior consists of sexual intercourse or needle sharing with a member of one of the high-risk groups.

Source: "Preventing the Heterosexual Spread of AIDS," Journal of the American Medical Association, April 22/29, 1988

fection and the onset of ARC (AIDS Related Complex) symptoms, which is four and one-half years, and a typical couple would have intercourse about 500 times during that period.

These risk estimates were based on approximate group averages. While individual risks may vary considerably, the researchers believe that the group estimates are not off by more than one order of magnitude. In this case, an order of magnitude is the difference between a number and that number multiplied by 10, for instance between 210 and 21. Risk groups and their prevalence are shown in the first two columns of the table. The value of 0.0001 for the prevalence of heterosexuals at low risk is based on data compiled from armed forces recruits and blood donors.

The prevalence listed for high risk groups varies from 0.05 to 0.5. Those at the higher end include homosexual/bisexual men and IV drug users from major metropolitan areas, and hemophiliacs. Hemophiliacs and others who received blood transfusions between 1978 and 1985 have a low risk in most parts of the country, but the risk jumps to as high as 1 percent per transfusion by the end of that time period in parts of the country with a high prevalence of AIDS and HIV infection. Unless these persons have been tested and proven seronegative, they should be considered high risk. Despite some recent findings concerning the inadequacies of blood testing for HIV infection, Drs. Hearst and Hulley maintain that those who received blood transfusions after 1985 are at extremely low risk due to the effectiveness of HIV testing in blood banks.

Those Who Test Negative

There are two categories for those who have tested negative for the HIV antibody: those who have no history of high risk behavior, i.e. neither homosexual or IV drug users, and those who test negative, but continue to participate in high risk behavior. The prevalence of infection among those who tested negative and are not engaged in high risk behavior depends on the accuracy of the antibody tests and the latency period between the time a person becomes infected and the time antibodies develop. The most commonly used commercially available test is ELISA (enzyme-linked immunosorbent assay) which is followed by a more precise Western blot study, which together have a sensitivity rate of

99 percent – only 1 in 100 persons who is really infected will get a negative result from the tests. The probability of infection in a person in a low-risk group who tested negative for HIV infection is 0.0001, but multiplied by the 1 percent false-negative rate for the antibody test, it becomes 0.00001.

For those who test negative, but continue high-risk behavior, the latency period discussed above is of great importance. Using an annual rate of 5 percent healthy, seronegative, high-risk individuals, and figuring an average of 10 weeks between the time of infection and the appearance of antibodies, the probability of being infected is 0.01. If reports that antibodies can take considerably longer to appear are true, then this estimation is too low.

The third column of the table, "Infectivity," reads the same for all categories: 0.002. This denotes the infectiveness of the virus which causes AIDS, HIV, or the risk of infection from one sexual contact with a person carrying the virus. Sexual contact for these purposes are defined as penile-vaginal intercourse with ejaculation. Most other forms of sexual activity carry with them either a considerably lower risk, or no risk at all.

Two alterable factors, however, which may increase infectivity are anal intercourse and the presence of genital ulcers. Another factor, which is not alterable, is the stage of the infection. It appears that the probability of the risk of infection increases as the disease progresses. The possibility also exists that certain genetic and anatomic characteristics of either partner, the strain of the virus, drug treatment, or other yet unknown factors may contribute to infectivity.

The Effectiveness of Condoms

The protective effectiveness of condoms is the final element in calculating the risk of infection. Condoms have a failure rate of 10 percent annually in preventing pregnancy, although some studies report better results. It is not known how often improper use, breakage, and slipping off, account for their failure. Information on the effectiveness of condoms in preventing pregnancy, however, is not particularly helpful in estimating their effectiveness in preventing HIV infection since pregnancy occurs only at ovulation.

A couple's motivation is undoubtedly a key factor in the effectiveness of condoms. For some couples, the prevention of AIDS may promote greater motivation for careful condom use than the prevention of pregnancy. For others who do not perceive the risk of infection, that may not be true. The study estimated that the use of condoms reduces the risk of infection by a factor of 10.

Implications

The primary factor for the extraordinary variation in the risk of HIV infection under various circumstances is the risk status of the sexual partner. Choosing a partner who is not in a high-risk group provides protection 5000-fold greater than that of choosing a partner in the highest-risk group. The use of condoms only provides one order of magnitude (a factor of 10), and a negative HIV antibody test provides only two orders of magnitude (a factor of 100) of protection.

The implications are obvious. The choice of sexual partners is more important today than it has ever been. A person must be certain that a potential partner is not in a high risk group and must be willing to go beyond asking that person about his past and present behavior. The person must get to know that person's friends and family to determine whether the answers are true. Sex with prostitutes, casual sex, and much of what is considered normal heterosexual behavior with someone other than an uninfected, steady partner is no longer smart nor advisable. Nothing prevents a person from lying about having had an HIV antibody test or about the results, although hiding membership in a high-risk group is more difficult.

EFFECTIVENESS OF PREVENTION VARIES

Limiting Partners

Limiting the number of sexual partners is effective when the partners are each less likely to be HIV carriers. People with numerous partners are less likely to really know their partners and to know if these partners are high-risk people or not. Promiscuous people (those who engage in sexual activity indiscriminantly) often choose promiscuous partners. While many partners can mean increased danger, fewer partners do not necessarily reverse the odds. A person must be careful that this smaller number of partners does not include members of high-risk groups. This is probably one of the most misunderstood aspects of AIDS education. Having sex with only one partner 100 times (a monogamous relationship for one year) who has a 1 percent chance of being infected carries nearly the same risk of having relations one time each with 100 different partners who average a 1 percent chance of being infected.

Using Condoms

While using condoms can reduce the risk of infection, the protection is not 100 percent. Even if condoms were more effective than they are, they would still be less effective than the careful choice of a partner. Use of a condom with an IV drug user, bisexual man, or prostitute places one at far greater risk than sex without a condom with someone who does not belong to any of these high-risk groups. If anything, the report expressed concern that the promotion of condoms may give some users who are in high-risk situations a false sense of security. In the case of partners, where one is known to be infected and the other is known not to be, Drs. Hearst and Hulley, believe the best advice would be to abstain, not to use condoms. Even with condoms, the uninfected partner has about a 1 in 11 chance of becoming infected after 500 encounters. On the other hand, condoms may not be necessary if sexual partners are not members of high risk groups. The risk of infection from an encounter with someone not in any high-risk group without a condom is about the same as being killed in a traffic accident while driving 10 miles to get to that encounter.

Avoiding Anal Intercourse

Evidence indicates that anal intercourse spreads HIV faster than vaginal intercourse, but, as with the use of condoms, is only high risk if done with a high-risk partner. Again, the choice of partners is the overwhelming factor.

MASTERS AND JOHNSON

In their recent book, CRISIS: Heterosexual Behavior in the Age of AIDS (1988, Grove Press), Dr. William H. Masters and Virginia E. Johnson, well-known and respected sex therapists, with Dr. Robert C. Kolodny, a medical researcher, analyzed the AIDS threat to the heterosexual population. Based on their own research findings, Masters and Johnson contend that AIDS is no longer confined to certain risk groups, but that undetected infections are significantly making their way into "straight" society and that authorities are drastically underestimating the number of those infected with AIDS. They also claim that neither intimate sexual contact nor sharing of intravenous drug needles is necessary for transmission of the virus. Transmission can occur when the blood or other body fluids from an infected person is splashed onto or rubbed against another person, if the previously uninfected person has a cut, rash, abrasion, broken blister, or some other weakness or opening in the skin. Recent CDC reports of rare instances of health care workers becoming infected would tend to bear this out. Masters and Johnson claim their goal in writing this book was not to frighten, but to motivate people to change their behavior.

Beginning in 1985, Masters and Johnson studied 800 sexually-active heterosexual adults between the ages of 21 and 40 who had 1.) no blood trans-fusion since 1977, 2.) no use of illicit drugs, and 3.) no homosexual or bi-sexual contact from 1977 to that time. The group was divided into two groups: 200 men and 200 women who said they were in a monogamous relationship (married or otherwise) for five years prior to the study; and 200 men and 200 women who admitted to at least 5 sex partners annually over the past five years. The study was conducted in New York, Los Angeles, St. Louis, and Atlanta. The first two cities are undisputed areas of high concentration of AIDS victims.

The researchers assumed those with a larger number of sex partners would be more likely to be infected with the AIDS virus than those with fewer sex partners. Couples were not recruited at random, but through church groups, childbirth classes, bulletin board announcements on college campuses, and fliers at single bars and dances. The nonmongamous women had an average number of 11.5 sex partners, while the men reported an average of 9.8 sex partners.

The prevalence of infection with the AIDS virus among the strictly monog-amous men and women was quite low. Only one of the 400 in that category, or 0.25 percent tested HIV-positive. Among those who reported multiple partners, the incidence of infection was considerably higher. Fourteen of the women (7 percent) and 10 men (5 percent) were infected with the virus. Among those who reported multiple partners, the subgroup which reported more than 12 partners a year had even higher prevalence - 14 percent of the women and 12 percent of the men tested positive. Not surprisingly, the highest percent of seropositive nonmonogamous subjects were found in New York and Los Angeles.

Fewer than 10 percent of those with multiple partners feared that they were exposing themselves to the AIDS virus. They believed that they would be able to recognize and avoid those who were in high risk groups. They were convinced, they claimed, that AIDS was not a threat to heterosexuals. None of the 200 multi-partner men reported using condoms regularly in the past year. Only 6 of the 200 women in this group routinely required their partners to use condoms when engaging in vaginal intercourse; four others asked their partners to use condoms during anal sex.

Masters and Johnson admit that because their sampling was not random and did not represent the overall population with respect to socio-economic status, education, and racial composition, they could not generalize their results (although they imply that by publishing their study). However, they feel their findings establish that AIDS has entrenched itself in the heterosexual communi-ty and that it will escalate at an alarming rate since heterosexuals with num-erous partners are most likely to be infected and estimate that 3 million Americans may already be infected, twice the number estimated by the CDC and other officials. The authors recommend mandatory virus testing for pregnant women, all those admitted to hospitals between ages 15 and 60, convicted pros-titutes and all those seeking a marriage license.

The Rebuttal

Most AIDS experts dispute the results of the study and question some of the conclusions the authors reached. While the experts agree that, under some circumstances, the risk to heterosexuals is great, there is still no evidence that the spread of the disease is rampant in the general population. Of the nearly 62,000 cases, 2,500, or 4 percent, were contracted through heterosexual intercourse, although officials expect that proportion to gradually rise. Officials believe the vast majority of these cases involve partners of IV drug users, bisexual men, or persons born in Africa or Haiti where heterosexual cases are far more common. Some AIDS researchers have found that, when questioned closely about their past contacts, heterosexuals eventually admit to past experience with drugs or homosexual activity, or have had sex partners who were in these high risk groups. Some experts have attacked the study for exaggerating the uncertain methods of transmission. Masters and Johnson indicated that transmission by mosquitoes and kissing should not be ruled out.

THE OTHER EXTREME

Many authorities believe the spread of AIDS might have been slowed sooner if gay leaders had closed the bathhouses much sooner since they were one of, if not the major sources of contact among gay men. Those who had fought the long, hard fight for gay sexual liberation were unwilling to relinquish the "freedom" of sexual expression which they had finally achieved. This attitude undoubtedly cost many thousands their lives. It is not surprising, then, that many who advocated sexual liberation for women would also look askance at warnings of the spread of AIDS into the heterosexual community and that limiting one's sexual activity and partners is an effective way to prevent its spread.

Helen Gurley Brown is editor and founder of Cosmopolitan magazine, a highly successful magazine with frequent articles about sexual fulfillment. Dr. Robert E. Gould, a clinical professor of both psychiatry and obstetrics and gynecology at New York Medical College, in "Reassuring News About AIDS: A Doctor Tells Why You May Not Be at Risk." (Cosmopolitan, January 1988) asserted that if the genitals of both heterosexual partners are intact and healthy, free from lesions or other infectious openings, then the HIV cannot be transmitted. Dr. Gould further claimed that vaginal secretions as well as other bodily fluids such as saliva and gastrointestinal have a neutralizing effect on the virus. Dr. Gould doubted reports of women who contracted AIDS in which the only risk factor was heterosexual intercourse with an infected partner. Many other physicians, including the head of the OB/GYN department where Dr. Gould teaches, do not endorse his findings.

Ms. Brown see AIDS as a mean of restoring guilt and celibacy to women who have just started to spread their sexual wings. She believes women will suffer more anxiety from the emotional upset of a cheating partner than by the fact he may bring home AIDS. Ms Brown also claims women cannot pass the virus on to other men. AIDS specialists, such as Dr. Redfield of the Walter Reed Army Institute describes AIDS as a "classical, sexually transmitted disease" which can be transmitted if placed on the mucous membranes of the vagina or the mouth.

Dr. Gould and Ms. Brown are not alone in their skepticism about the spread of AIDS into the heterosexual community, just as Masters and Johnson are not alone in their position. Cosmopolitan is a very popular periodical and the sex therapists are very well-respected in their fields and well-known among the general public. There may well be some truth in each of their positions. The important thing is that the public must learn about AIDS information as it comes out and become critically aware in spite of the fact that, as Dr. Redfield points out, "most people want to believe those who tell us not to worry."

CHAPTER VI

THOSE WITH NO FUTURE - CHILDREN WITH AIDS

Children with AIDS had no control over their infection with this deadly disease. They were simply born to the wrong person at the wrong time or had the wrong disease that required transfusions. Children and youth with AIDS are a growing number who require special help.

DIFFERS FROM ADULT AIDS

The same virus, human immunodeficiency virus (HIV), causes AIDS in both adults and children by attacking and damaging their immune and central nervous systems. However, The development and the course of the disease differ considerably.

It is particularly difficult to detect the AIDS virus in infants because HIV-infected mothers may transmit the antibodies as well as the virus to their babies. Infants who show a positive result on the antibody test at birth, may later test negative, indicating that the mother transmitted the HIV antibodies, but not the virus itself. (Remember the antibody test does not directly show HIV infection, but rather the presence of antibodies to the virus).

In adults, symptoms of fully developed AIDS include the presence of opportunistic infections and/or rare cancers, and most adult deaths are caused by these diseases. The most common are Pneumocystis carinii pneumonia, a rare pneumonia, and Kaposi's sarcoma, a rare skin cancer that can spread to internal organs. As many as 80 percent of AIDS patients have had one or both of these conditions. Other disorders found in adult AIDS patients are leukemia-like cancer, prolonged diarrhea causing severe dehydration, weight loss, and central nervous system infections that can lead to dementia.

Among infants and children, the disease is more often characterized by failure to thrive and unusually severe bacterial infections. With the exception of Pneumocystis carinii pneumonia, children with symptomatic HIV infection do not often develop frequent and diverse opportunistic infections like adults. More often, they are plagued by recurrent bacterial infections, persistent or recurrent oral thrush (a common fungal infection of the mouth or throat), and chronic or recurrent diarrhea. They may also suffer from enlarged lymph nodes, chronic pneumonia, developmental delays, and neurologic abnormalities.

A DEFINITION FOR CHILDREN

Although the Centers for Disease Control updated the CDC surveillance definition for AIDS in 1987, there was still no standard definitions for other

HIV characteristics found in children. Physicians who worked with large numbers of HIV-infected children reported that only about half of their patients met the criteria of the CDC surveillance definition for AIDS. The CDC convened a panel of consultants and published their definition in the April 24, 1987 Morbidity and Mortality Weekly Report.

The HIV infection in children is primarily identified by the presence of the virus in the blood or tissues, ideally confirmed by culture or other laboratory techniques. Detection of the antibody in most adults has been identified by a culture, to determine infection, but similar studies involving children have not been reported. In addition, infants may carry a passively (undetected) transferred antibody from the mother which limits interpretation of a positive antibody test. Most of those involved in this research believed this passively transferred HIV antibody could sometimes exist for up to 15 months. Therefore two definitions were needed: one for infants and children up to 15 months of age who were exposed to their infection perinatally, and another definition for older children with perinatal infection and for infants and children of all ages acquiring the virus through other means.

Under 15 months

Infection in those infants and children who are under 15 months and were exposed to their infected mothers perinatally can be defined by one or more of the following symptoms: 1) identification of the virus in blood or tissues; 2) the presence of HIV antibody indicated by testing and evidence of both humoral and cellular immune deficiency, as well as meeting the requirements for one or more categories in Class P-2 (see accompanying table of HIV definition); 3) symptoms meeting the previously published definition for AIDS. Infants and children who were perinatally exposed who lack one of the criteria should be observed further for HIV-related illness and tested at regular intervals. Those who later test virus-culture negative, and continue to have no confirmed normalities associated with HIV infection, are unlikely to be infected.

The CDC believes that HIV infection in perinatally exposed infants and children under 15 months can be difficult to diagnose. Those who are HIV-seropositive and are asymptomatic (without symptoms) without immune abnormalities have an HIV infection status which cannot be determined unless virus culture or other antigen-detection tests are positive. A negative culture does not necessarily mean no infection, since the sensitivity of the culture may be low. Overall, the pattern of HIV-infection in infants is not well defined.

Older Children

HIV infection in older children is defined by one or more of the following: 1) identification of the virus in the blood or tissues; 2) the presence of HIV antibody (positive screening plus confirmatory test) regardless of the presence of immunologic abnormalities or signs or symptoms; or 3) confirmation that symptoms meet the previously published CDC case definition for AIDS.

HOW MANY?

The Centers for Disease Control (CDC) in Atlanta reported that by May 23, 1988, 990 cases of AIDS in children (those under age 13 at time of diagnosis) had been reported since record-keeping began in 1981. Of those, 53 percent (524) were black, and 22 percent (222) were Hispanic. The remainder were white, with the exception of the 1 percent whose racial/ethnic background was unknown. Of these 990, 580 have died since 1981.

Summary of the definition of HIV infection in children

Infants and children under 15 months of age with perinatal infection

1) Virus in blood or tissues
   or
2) HIV antibody
   and
   evidence of both cellular and humoral immune deficiency
   and
   one or more categories in Class P-2
   or
3) Symptoms meeting CDC case definition for AIDS

Older children with perinatal infection and children with HIV infection acquired through other modes of transmission

1) Virus in blood or tissues
   or
2) HIV antibody
   or
3) Symptoms meeting CDC case definition for AIDS

Summary of the classification of HIV infection in children under 13 years of age

Class P-0. Indeterminate infection

Class P-1. Asymptomatic infection

    Subclass A. Normal immune function
    Subclass B. Abnormal immune function
    Subclass C. Immune function not tested

Class P-2. Symptomatic infection

    Subclass A. Nonspecific findings
    Subclass B. Progressive neurologic disease
    Subclass C. Lymphoid interstitial pneumonitis
    Subclass D. Secondary infectious diseases
      Category D-1. Specified secondary infectious diseases listed in the CDC surveillance definition for AIDS
      Category D-2. Recurrent serious bacterial infections
      Category D-3. Other specified secondary infectious diseases
    Subclass E. Secondary cancers
      Category E-1. Specified secondary cancers listed in the CDC surveillance definition for AIDS
      Category E-2. Other cancers possibly secondary to HIV infection
    Subclass F. Other diseases possibly due to HIV infection

Source: Reports on AIDS, June 1986-May 1987, Centers for Disease Control, (WDC, 1987)

GEOGRAPHY

The geography of AIDS in children is consistent with that of AIDS resulting from intravenous drug abuse and among Haitian immigrants. States with a high incidence of IV-associated AIDS, New York, New Jersey, (these two states account for 75 percent of AIDS cases in IV drug users) and Florida, also have high rates of children with AIDS. Florida and New York are home to 79 percent of all Haitian immigrants. In late May 1988, over 31 percent of the childhood cases of AIDS were reported in New York, 13 percent in New Jersey, and almost 12 percent in Florida. (For a state by state breakdown for AIDS among children, see page 25.)

The proportion of AIDS cases among children reported from states other than the three mentioned above increased from 24 percent in 1982-1984 to 34 percent in 1985-1986. By mid-1988, 44 percent of the reports were from other states and territories. This is consistent with a U.S. Health Department estimate that by 1991, 80 percent of all AIDS cases would occur outside of New York City and San Francisco, the cities hardest hit thus far.

TRANSMISSION CATEGORIES[2]

ADULTS/ADOLESCENTS	MALES				FEMALES				TOTAL			
	Since Jan 1		Cumulative		Since Jan 1		Cumulative		Since Jan 1		Cumulative	
	Number	(%)	Number	(%)	Number	(%)	Number	(%)	Number	(%)	Number	(%)
Homosexual/Bisexual Male	6772	(62)	39001	(69)					6772	(56)	39001	(63)
Intravenous (IV) Drug Abuser	2283	(21)	8978	(16)	686	(54)	2546	(52)	2969	(24)	11524	(19)
Homosexual Male and IV Drug Abuser	800	(7)	4568	(8)					800	(7)	4568	(7)
Hemophilia/Coagulation Disorder	122	(1)	585	(1)	3	(0)	21	(0)	125	(1)	606	(1)
Heterosexual Cases[3]	206	(2)	1120	(2)	311	(25)	1415	(29)	517	(4)	2535	(4)
Transfusion, Blood/Components	227	(2)	990	(2)	137	(11)	537	(11)	364	(3)	1527	(2)
Undetermined[4]	485	(4)	1578	(3)	122	(10)	411	(8)	607	(5)	1989	(3)
SUBTOTAL [% of all cases]	10895	[90]	56820	[92]	1259	[10]	4930	[8]	12154	[100]	61750	[100]
CHILDREN[5]												
Hemophilia/Coagulation Disorder	14	(11)	53	(10)	1	(1)	3	(1)	15	(6)	56	(6)
Parent with/at risk of AIDS[6]	91	(68)	384	(71)	84	(85)	378	(84)	175	(75)	762	(77)
Transfusion, Blood/Components	23	(17)	84	(16)	10	(10)	50	(11)	33	(14)	134	(14)
Undetermined[4]	5	(4)	19	(4)	4	(4)	19	(4)	9	(4)	38	(4)
SUBTOTAL [% of all cases]	133	[57]	540	[55]	99	[43]	450	[45]	232	[100]	990	[100]
TOTAL [% of all cases]	11028	[89]	57360	[91]	1358	[11]	5380	[9]	12386	[100]	62740[7]	[100]

For notes on the above table, see notes below the top table on following page.

AGE AT DIAGNOSIS BY RACIAL/ETHNIC GROUP

AGE GROUP	WHITE, NOT HISPANIC		BLACK, NOT HISPANIC		HISPANIC		OTHER[5]/ UNKNOWN		TOTAL	
	Cumulative		Cumulative		Cumulative		Cumulative		Cumulative	
	Number	(%)	Number	(%)	Number	(%)	Number	(%)	Number	(%)
Under 5	159	(0)	469	(3)	197	(2)	8	(1)	833	(1)
5 - 12	75	(0)	55	(0)	25	(0)	2	(0)	157	(0)
13 - 19	125	(0)	89	(1)	46	(1)	5	(1)	265	(0)
20 - 29	6984	(19)	3787	(23)	2102	(23)	104	(18)	12977	(21)
30 - 39	16722	(45)	7851	(48)	4250	(47)	254	(43)	29077	(46)
40 - 49	8309	(23)	2820	(17)	1754	(19)	142	(24)	13025	(21)
Over 49	4449	(12)	1211	(7)	676	(7)	70	(12)	6406	(10)
TOTAL [% OF ALL CASES]	36823	[59]	16282	[26]	9050	[14]	585	[1]	62740	[100]

[5] Includes patients whose race/ethnicity is Asian/Pacific Islander (367 persons) and American Indian/Alaskan Native (64 persons).

Source: "AIDS Weekly Surveillance Report," Centers for Disease Control, May 23, 1988

A CONGRESSIONAL REPORT

The House Select Committee on Children, Youth, and Families has done considerable research and held numerous hearings on the issue of children and AIDS. The Committee reported its findings in A Generation in Jeopardy: Children and AIDS (100th Congress, 1st Session December 1987).

Alarming Rise

During the first 11 months of 1987, the number of reported AIDS cases among infants and children rose more than 60 percent. By November 1987, 691 cases of children under 13 with AIDS had been reported, up by at least 271 cases from January 1987. (A May 23, 1988 tally showed 990 cases, up 300 cases or 43 percent in six months).

Although reported childhood AIDS cases represent fewer than 2 percent of all diagnosed AIDS cases, many experts believe cases of both adults and children are underreported. In May 21, 1986 testimony before the House Select Committee, Dr. James Oleske of the University of Medicine and Dentistry of New Jersey, an institution which has seen a large number of childhood AIDS cases, testified that the 350 cases which had been reported to the CDC at that time severely underreported the actual number, which he estimated to be closer to 2,000 cases. Other experts in the field agree. In addition to those with undisputed cases of pediatric AIDS, many more children are thought to be infected, but asymptomatic.

TRANSMISSION CATEGORIES BY RACIAL/ETHNIC GROUP	WHITE, NOT HISPANIC Cumulative Number (%)		BLACK, NOT HISPANIC Cumulative Number (%)		HISPANIC Cumulative Number (%)		OTHER[8]/ UNKNOWN Cumulative Number (%)		TOTAL Cumulative Number (%)	
ADULTS/ADOLESCENTS										
Homosexual/Bisexual Male	28710	(78)	6010	(38)	3891	(44)	390	(68)	39001	(63)
Intravenous (IV) Drug Abuser	2229	(6)	5846	(37)	3392	(38)	57	(10)	11524	(19)
Homosexual Male and IV Drug Abuser	2796	(8)	1111	(7)	638	(7)	23	(4)	4568	(7)
Hemophilia/Coagulation Disorder	513	(1)	41	(0)	40	(0)	12	(2)	606	(1)
Heterosexual Cases[3]	458	(1)	1723	(11)	342	(4)	12	(2)	2535	(4)
Transfusion, Blood/Components	1136	(3)	234	(1)	119	(1)	38	(7)	1527	(2)
Undetermined[4]	747	(2)	793	(5)	406	(5)	43	(7)	1989	(3)
SUBTOTAL [% of all cases]	36589	[59]	15758	[26]	8828	[14]	575	[1]	61750	[100]
CHILDREN[5]										
Hemophilia/Coagulation Disorder	41	(18)	6	(1)	7	(3)	2	(20)	56	(6)
Parent with/at risk of AIDS[6]	111	(47)	464	(89)	180	(81)	7	(70)	762	(77)
Transfusion, Blood/Components	75	(32)	31	(6)	27	(12)	1	(10)	134	(14)
Undetermined[4]	7	(3)	23	(4)	8	(4)			38	(4)
SUBTOTAL [% of all cases]	234	[24]	524	[53]	222	[22]	10	[1]	990	[100]
TOTAL [% of all cases]	36823	[59]	16282	[26]	9050	[14]	585	[1]	62740[7]	[100]

[1] These data are provisional.

[2] Cases with more than one risk factor other than the combinations listed in the tables or footnotes are tabulated only in the category listed first.

[3] Includes 1518 persons (327 men, 1191 women) who have had heterosexual contact with a person with AIDS or at risk for AIDS and 1017 persons (793 men, 224 women) without other identified risks who were born in countries in which heterosexual transmission is believed to play a major role although precise means of transmission have not yet been fully defined.

[4] Includes patients on whom risk information is incomplete (due to death, refusal to be interviewed or loss to follow-up), patients still under investigation, men reported only to have had heterosexual contact with a prostitute, and interviewed patients for whom no specific risk was identified; also includes one health-care worker who seroconverted to HIV and developed AIDS after documented needlestick to blood.

[5] Includes all patients under 13 years of age at time of diagnosis.

[6] Epidemiologic data suggest transmission from an infected mother to her fetus or infant during the perinatal period.

[7] Includes 6457 patients who meet only the 1987 revised surveillance definition for AIDS.

[8] Includes patients whose race/ethnicity is Asian/Pacific Islander (367 persons) and American Indian/Alaskan Native (64 persons).

AIDS CASES BY TRANSMISSION CATEGORIES AND DATE OF REPORT TO CDC, TWELVE-MONTH TOTALS

TRANSMISSION CATEGORIES[1]	Year Ending MAY 23, 1987 Number (%)		Year Ending MAY 23, 1988 Number (%)		CUMULATIVE CASES AND DEATHS SINCE JUNE 1981 Number (%)		Deaths	(% Cases)
ADULTS/ADOLESCENTS								
Homosexual/Bisexual Male	9985	(66.3)	15481	(59.4)	39001	(63.2)	21661	(62.6)
Intravenous (IV) Drug Abuser	2406	(16.0)	5485	(21.0)	11524	(18.7)	6396	(18.5)
Homosexual Male and IV Drug Abuser	1087	(7.2)	1825	(7.0)	4568	(7.4)	2731	(7.9)
Hemophilia/Coagulation Disorder	175	(1.2)	261	(1.0)	606	(1.0)	357	(1.0)
Heterosexual Cases[2]	604	(4.0)	1112	(4.3)	2535	(4.1)	1358	(3.9)
Transfusion, Blood/Components	395	(2.6)	790	(3.0)	1527	(2.5)	1032	(3.0)
Undetermined[3]	412	(2.7)	1111	(4.3)	1989	(3.2)	1073	(3.1)
SUBTOTAL	15064	(100.0)	26065	(100.0)	61750	(100.0)	34608	(100.0)
CHILDREN[4]								
Hemophilia/Coagulation Disorder	14	(6.2)	29	(6.2)	56	(5.7)	34	(5.9)
Parent with/at risk of AIDS[5]	186	(81.9)	349	(74.7)	762	(77.0)	441	(76.0)
Transfusion, Blood/Components	21	(9.3)	66	(14.1)	134	(13.5)	82	(14.1)
Undetermined[3]	6	(2.6)	23	(4.9)	38	(3.8)	23	(4.0)
SUBTOTAL	227	(100.0)	467	(100.0)	990	(100.0)	580	(100.0)
TOTAL	15291		26532		62740		35188	

[1] Cases with more than one risk factor other than the combinations listed in the tables or footnotes are tabulated only in the category listed first.

[2] Includes 1518 persons (327 men, 1191 women) who have had heterosexual contact with a person with AIDS or at risk for AIDS and 1017 persons (793 men, 224 women) without other identified risks who were born in countries in which heterosexual transmission is believed to play a major role although precise means of transmission have not yet been fully defined.

[3] Includes patients on whom risk information is incomplete (due to death, refusal to be interviewed or loss to follow-up), patients still under investigation, men reported only to have had heterosexual contact with a prostitute, and interviewed patients for whom no specific risk was identified; also includes one health-care worker who seroconverted to HIV and developed AIDS after documented needlestick to blood.

[4] Includes all patients under 13 years of age at time of diagnosis.

[5] Epidemiologic data suggest transmission from an infected mother to her fetus or infant during the perinatal period.

[6] This table cumulates cases by DATE OF DIAGNOSIS rather than DATE OF REPORT. Because of this difference, totals may differ from those in other tables and will change with late reports and new data or information. Data are provided for the 20 SMSA's currently reporting the largest number of AIDS cases.

Source: "AIDS Weekly Surveillance Report,"
Centers for Disease Control, May 23, 1988

Until the recent CDC definition specifically designed for children (described above), children needed a specific indication of being immune-deficient, such as an opportunistic infection, and no other disease which could cause immune deficiency. Because many children did not meet the previously strict definition, they were not reported. Some pediatricians believe there are three to five times as many children with (ARC) Aids Related Complex as there are cases of AIDS. In addition, some researchers in New York, the home of the largest incidence of AIDS in children, estimate that within the next two to three years, 20-25 percent of children with ARC will develop an opportunistic infection and consequently, AIDS.

It Won't Get Any Better

There is every indication the increase in the number children with AIDS will continue. The Surgeon General of the United States, C. Everett Koop, in Report of the Surgeon General's Workshop on Children with HIV Infection and Their Families (WDC, 1987) estimated that by 1991 the number of children with AIDS will have increased to 3,000, and virtually all will die within three years. This is an increase of about 300 percent from the May 1988 number, and, according to Dr. Koop, "is undoubtedly underestimated."

The National Commission to Prevent Infant Mortality, in Perinatal AIDS (WDC, 1987), reports that some cities are expecting more cases of AIDS than is officially predicated. Department of Health officials in New York City expect as many as 4,000 cases of AIDS by 1991. The Washington D.C. Mayor's Task Force on AIDS projects over 1,000 cases for their city alone. The New Jersey Department of Health reported a 400 percent increase in the number of pediatric cases from 1986-1987 and sees no reason why this rate of increase will not continue.

Perinatal Transmission

The expected increase is based on the growing numbers of women in their childbearing years who are infected with HIV. Of the more than 3,300 cases of AIDS in women reported by November 1987, 97 percent were of childbearing age. A report by two CDC scientists based on November 1986 figures, found that of the 1,819 women infected at that time, 79 percent were between ages 13 and 39. (See Chapter V). Either proportion is frightening when remembering that about 80 percent of AIDS cases in children occur perinatally. If the projected estimate of 20,000 women of childbearing age with AIDS by 1991 becomes reality, the consequences for their children can be horrible.

Dr. Lorraine Hale, executive director of the Hale House in New York City, which for many years has provided a group home environment for babies born to drug addicted mothers, speaking before the Select Committee on Narcotics Abuse and Control, U.S. House of Representatives (July 27, 1987), described the enormity of the problem.

Ten years ago, it was estimated that in New York State, there were 28,000 female users, 26,000 of childbearing age, [each] capable of giving birth to 3.5 babies over a 15 year period. Given today's statistics, we find there are 75,000 women in methadone maintenance programs. Sixty-three percent or 47,250 have positive antibodies for the AIDS virus. They too are each capable of giving birth to 3.5 babies over a 15 year period, for a total of 165,375 babies, the vast majority of whom will also test positive for the antibodies.

Experts now estimate that approximately 50,000 women in New York City are infected, but asymptomatic, and most of them unaware. These women are 3 percent of the city's childbearing-age women. Some researchers estimate an infection rate of 50 percent for New York City women drug users, and 20 percent among those whose sexual partners are addicts. Reports from drug counselors in New York City in late June 1988 indicate that those who use crack, the highly-addictive smokable form of cocaine, are also becoming increasingly more at risk for infection. Crack houses, which can be found in large numbers in many urban areas (as well as some suburban and rural areas), are places where many people gather to smoke crack. Often, group sex takes place, since the binge smoking of crack can heighten sexual arousal as well as lower inhibitions. Having multiple sexual partners make encountering a partner with the AIDS virus more likely, in addition to giving the virus more opportunity to infect.

Unfortunately, it is difficult to fully determine how infected mothers transmit the virus to their babies. One Public Health study found that 50 percent of mothers who had delivered one infected baby, also transmitted the virus to later children. The CDC estimates that one-third of infected mothers will give birth to infected infants. Experts believe transmission could occur during pregnancy, through the placenta; during labor and delivery, through exposure to maternal blood and vaginal secretions; or after birth through breast feeding, but at this point no one is sure.

Other Means of Transmittal

Among children under age 13 with AIDS, 77 percent had a parent infected with AIDS; 14 percent received a contaminated transfusion; 6 percent regularly received blood products because of a hemophilia/coagulation disorder; while 4 percent were of an undetermined origin. Several physicians and social workers have reported a small number of children infected as a result of sexual molestation and abuse, but because very little research has been done in the area of transmission due to sexual abuse, there is no way to tell how prevalent it is.

Children who live in environments where intravenous drug use is common are also potentially exposed to contaminated needles. One 9-year-old in New York City who first showed signs of AIDS symptoms at age 7 is believed to have contracted AIDS from playing with her parent's contaminated needles.

Most Have Died

Almost 60 percent of all children diagnosed with AIDS have died. Of those diagnosed before 1984, 75-80 percent have died, according to Dr. Oleske. As with reporting of all AIDS data, deaths involving AIDS are also likely to be underreported. The life span for infants with AIDS (not just the HIV infection, or ARC) is about one year after diagnosis, although this can vary. The final mortality rate for infected children is also not known.

Minority Children Hit Hard

The CDC reports that 75 percent of all children with AIDS are either black or Hispanic. These are often children who already face substantial obstacles of poor health, poverty, lack of adequate care, and fewer educational advantages. Minorities compose only one-fifth of the U.S. population, but account for two-fifths of the reported AIDS cases with minority women and children facing the greatest risks.

As of May 23, 1988, 53 percent (524) of the children under age 13 with AIDS were black; 22 percent (222) were Hispanic; 24 percent (234) were white; and 1 percent (10) were of other or unknown races. Black children make up only 15 percent of the U.S. population of children, and Hispanic children only 10 percent. Eighty-six percent of the minority children with AIDS and 47 percent of white children were infected perinatally.

WHO WILL CARE FOR THEM AND HOW?

Children with AIDS face multiple and devastating health problems. Not only are they plagued by pneumonia, swollen lymph organs, and chronic diarrhea, but about half have an encephalopathy (a disease of the brain), which further complicates treatment and rehabilitation. Those who specialize in such care say treatment programs are "catch-as-catch-can," without organized support in areas where the concentration of patients is the heaviest. Dr. Oleske reports that specific therapy programs which deal with both the overwhelming physical and psychological issues these children face are unavailable. Many facilities attempt to provide rehabilitation, but because of the children's multiple problems including the brain disorders and their deprived backgrounds, these children are still not getting the quality of care they need.

Most children with AIDS come from poor families which means they are likely to receive their care at public hospitals, which as Dr. Margaret Heagarty of Harlem Hospital in NYC notes, "almost by definition are embattled institutions that survive hand to mouth." The AIDS epidemic has added further strain to hospitals which were already barely surviving economically. She further points out that not only is the care of AIDS patients inadequate, but the entire municipal health care system is threatened by the huge expense involved in treating AIDS patients.

Testifying before the House Select Committee on Children, Youth, and Families (February 21, 1987), William Barrick, R.N., M.S.N., with the AIDS Project in Berkeley, California, was certain that the demand for care for these children would increase dramatically.

Infant services will be seeing unknown numbers of children with chronic and mortal disease. The danger of live-virus immunization of children with AIDS may cause such diseases as measles, rubella, and mumps to reappear among these children. Frequent office visits to pediatricians for close follow-up will become routine. In-patient treatment of infections will be far more frequent on this group. Acute care hospital admissions for diagnosis and treatment of neurological manifestations of AIDS will be more frequent.

In addition, the hospital staff who care for children with AIDS will require special training in order to understand the disease and the appropriate care. Just as importantly, they will need to know how to protect themselves from HIV infection.

Abandoned and Orphaned

For many young victims of AIDS who have been abandoned by their parents, hospitals and social service agencies have become substitutes for homes. Some of these babies already have AIDS or test positive for HIV with no signs yet of the illness. Many children who are not clinically ill are staying in hospitals for lack of adequate placement, especially in heavily concentrated areas like New York City. The cost of the extended, but unnecessary, hospitalization of these "boarder babies," as they have come to be called, has been great. Considering the first 37 children with AIDS cared for by Harlem Hospital, 30 percent of the hospital days and 20 percent of the total cost were not medically necessary, but could not be avoided because these was no where else to send the children.

The situation has been eased somewhat by the development of specialized foster care, long sought by physicians and other health care workers. In July 1987, some 30 children with AIDS had been orphaned or abandoned and were being boarded in New York City hospitals while awaiting foster families. In some cases, when children had been placed in foster care prior to the AIDS diagnosis, foster parents left the children in hospitals after the diagnosis because they could not or would not cope with the physical, emotional, and financial burdens such care entailed.

In addition to their physical problems, many children with AIDS who have been abandoned experience the fear, isolation, and psychological scars common to the terminally and chronically ill. The absence of consistent one-on-one care can cause emotional disturbances, as well as developmental delays. Very often these children seem more like emotionally disturbed than physically sick children. A spokesman for a day-care center for AIDS children in Bronx, New York, reported that these children could not distinguish between day and night or between friends and strangers. They lack a sense of cause and effect, and of what a day is or when things should be done. They find transitions difficult.

Efforts Promising, but Few

Areas such as New York City, which has the greatest numbers of pediatric AIDS cases, have responded with new specialized services offering promise of better treatment and care. At Albert Einstein Medical Center, in the Bronx, New York, an institution in the forefront of care for children with AIDS, a comprehensive clinic, including a mother's support group has served over 200 children with AIDS. New York City also has a city-financed day care center in the Bronx where 35 percent of the city's pediatric AIDS cases are being taken care of. Children's Hospital in Newark, New Jersey has an early intervention program and offers support to families that has helped reduce the mortality rate among the children and improved the quality of their lives by reducing the number of recurring serious infections. New York has two private foster care agencies specially designed to find homes for AIDS children, including offering more than twice the financial support ordinarily received for foster care reimbursements. The recently-opened Hale House Cradle is to provide care for unrelated babies born addicted to drugs who also test positive for antibodies to the AIDS virus. A similar home, St. Clair's in Elizabeth, New Jersey, has been operating since May 1987.

THE COST - HIGH AND GETTING HIGHER

Perinatal AIDS (1987), a study conducted by the National Commission to Prevent Infant Mortality, found that it cost Harlem Hospital in New York City $3.4 million worth of in-hospital costs alone to treat 37 children with AIDS or positive HIV. The 37 young patients had 6,035 in-hospital patient days ranging from $300-$2,400 per day. Dr. Hale, of Harlem Hospital and Hale House Cradle, reported that monitoring one baby for one day costs $600, or $219,000 per year. The hospital care of Hale House Cradle will cost about $161 per day, or $58,765 per year. Medicare will cover these children in homes or in hospitals.

The U.S. Health and Human Services Department has estimated that, given current trends in the number of children and adult AIDS cases and the cost of medical treatment, the estimated cost for hospital as well as out-patient medical care for AIDS by 1991 will be $8 billion, although costs could go as high as $18 billion.

ADOLESCENTS AND AIDS - A TICKING BOMB

Presently, the number of AIDS cases among adolescents has been low. As of June 27, 1988 CDC reported 273 cases among 13-19-year-olds, about 0.4 percent of the total 65,780 cases cases reported. Of these cases among teens, about 45 percent were white, 34 percent, black, 18 percent, Hispanic, and 3 percent were of other or unknown races. There were 13,643 cases among 20-29-year-olds, about 21 percent of reported AIDS cases. Due to the typically long latency period between becoming infected and onset of symptoms, it is highly probable that many in the latter age group became infected as teenagers. AIDS cases among teens were clustered in New Jersey, New York, and Florida.

At Special Risk

The transmission and course of HIV infection among adolescents is more like that among adult cases than among infants and children. Adolescents are infected primarily through receipt of contaminated blood and blood products, sexual activity with an infected partner, and drug abuse using contaminated needles.

The characteristics of adolescence as a time for development, uncertainty, and a false sense of invulnerability creates the potential for young people to become particularly vulnerable to HIV infection. This is a time of experimentation, often in terms of sexual behavior or use of illicit drugs.

Gay and lesbian youth, struggling with their sexuality, may engage in homosexual encounters far away from home, but maintain and engage in heterosexual relationships in their neighborhoods to avoid suspicion. Delinquents, runaways, homeless youth, and victims of child abuse are more at risk to exposure to the AIDS virus, because they are more likely to be involved in sexual experimentation, prostitution, and drug use.

Most are Sexually Active

Numerous studies have shown that approximately 70 percent of girls and 80 percent of boys have engaged in sexual intercourse at least once by the time they are 20 years old. Although the pregnancy rate among American teenagers has been declining recently, there are one million teen pregnancies annually.

Engaging in sexual activity before sufficient maturity, coupled with ineffective contraceptive methods, has given sexually active teenagers the highest rate of sexually transmitted diseases (STD) among heterosexuals of all age groups. Conservative estimates indicate that one out of seven teens currently has an STD - approximately 2.5 million teenagers are affected by STD each year. The most prevalent are chlamydia and gonorrhea. Fewer than 20 percent of sexually active girls 15-19 years-old reported using a barrier type contraceptive (condoms or diaphragms) which afford some protection against STD, including AIDS. Surgeon General Koop reported that the National Survey of Family Growth found that about half of teenagers used some form of contraceptive at first intercourse (this is one of the more positive estimates), and that those who did, tended to use condoms. The younger the teen, the more likely the person was to use a condom than other methods, no doubt due to their easy availability and their relatively low cost. Condom use appears to be a teachable technique for sexually active adolescents, although abstinence is the preferred technique.

Heterosexual Transmission Rising

A high rate of sexual activity among teens, plus the highest rates of STD, can mean extreme vulnerability to heterosexually transmitted AIDS. A recent study ("Pace of Heterosexual AIDS Spread Surprise Scientists," Washington Post October 6, 1987) of over 4,000 patients treated at an inner-city STD clinic, found that 6.3 percent of the men and 3 percent of the women were HIV-infected. Of those, one-third of the males and half of the females were infected through heterosexual activity.

The rise in the heterosexual transmission of AIDS is best shown by the changing male to female ratio of AIDS infection. For all ages, in the U.S., the male to female ratio is 12:1, due to the greater number of AIDS cases among homosexual males. Evidence suggests that the concentration of the infection among homosexual males may be leveling off or declining. Simultaneously, the rate is increasing among other risk groups, such as IV drug users, their sexual partners, and their offspring.

Among adolescent AIDS cases in New York City, the male to female ratio is 2.8:1, suggesting increased heterosexual transmission. A September 1987 study of 118 New York youth ages 13 to 21, infected with AIDS, most of whom were Hispanic and black, showed a significantly lower incidence of homosexuality or bisexuality (44 percent) compared to adults (66 percent), but a higher percentage were IV drug abusers (23 percent compared to 16 percent of all adults) or female partners of these two groups (11 percent compared to 2 percent). Slightly less than 20 percent of the New York City male adolescent AIDS cases were transfusion recipients or hemophiliacs, as compared to 80 percent of younger adolescent males in other parts of the country.

Minority Teens at High Risk

Minority teens have a higher prevalence of STD and are more likely to be living in poverty, placing them at greater risk for AIDS. This heightened risk comes at a time when the proportion of minority youth in this country is rising rapidly. At present, of the more than 35 million youth ages 10-19 in the U.S., more than 6 million are minorities. Over the next 10 years, the adolescent population is expected to increase by about 10 percent, with the bulk of the increases occurring in the West and Southwest. Ethnic minorities, particularly Hispanic and Asian youth will make up the largest increases in adolescent population. The Hispanic community in many areas has been hit quite hard by the AIDS epidemic, while the Asian community has not.

Minorities have a far greater incidence of STD than their white counterparts. The average age-adjusted gonorrhea rate among black males aged 15-19 years is about 15 times that of their white peers, while the rate for black females in the same age group is 10 times that for white females. Young black females had the highest rate of chlamydia (23 percent); young Hispanic females, 14 percent; young white females, 10 percent.

Hemophilia-Associated AIDS

From 1982, when the first cases of AIDS in hemophiliacs were reported through October 1987, 57 out the 184 teenage AIDs cases (31 percent) involved teens with hemophilia (a hereditary disease in which normal clotting factors are lacking, so the blood does not clot). Adolescent hemophiliacs were 13 percent of the total of 440 hemophilia-associated AIDS cases at that time. Nationally, 80 percent of the 11-17 year-old male adolescents with AIDS are hemophiliacs. (While females may help carry hemophilia from generation to generation, only males get hemophilia.) About one-quarter of all hemophiliac-associated AIDS cases involved 20-29 year olds.

The latest statistics show that two-thirds of all hemophiliacs are sero-positive for HIV. Depending on the type of clotting factor they received, 22-75 percent of hemophiliacs have tested positive for AIDS antibodies. It is hoped that improved testing of the blood supply (and the blood clotting factor) will prevent the virus from being transmitted this way in the future.

Researchers estimate that 15-17 percent of sexual partners of hemophiliacs with AIDS are now infected themselves. Although 98 percent of hemophiliacs who responded to a recent study had acquired the essential facts about the transmission of AIDS, 50 percent did not practice "safe sex". This lack of more careful sexual practices is especially dangerous among adolescents, 60 percent of whom experience tongue kissing (while saliva in small amounts is not known to be dangerous, deep kissing of an infected person is discouraged) and for whom the use of condoms is not popular.

At Long Island Jewish Medical Center in New Hyde Park, New York, professionals who treat and counsel young men with hemophilia, often find the questions from their young, hemophiliac patients hard to answer. Should they date and have sexual relations? Should they tell their dates they may be carrying the AIDS virus? Most wonder if they will ever have any kind of a relationship. Professionals are advised to be neutral in their counseling, and present detailed information about safer sex (cautioning that condoms are not foolproof), and suggest they bring their girlfriends to counseling sessions. This neutrality is difficult for the counselors who can never be sure if these young men are infecting their partners. The young men are often torn and indecisive, searching for concrete answers that may not exist and probably would not be easy, if they did.

Drug Use and Adolescents

Recent studies indicate that about 1 percent of high school seniors reported having used heroin, almost 17 percent reported having ever used cocaine, and 23 percent reported having used stimulants. All of these drugs can be taken intravenously. Teenagers are less likely than adults to inject drugs, but those who do and use shared needles are at an increased risk for infection with the AIDS virus. This is particularly true of those who are considered "street youth" and are more likely to be exposed to high risk behavior. The number of youths using IV drugs outside of urban areas seems to be relatively low, but suburban athletes have been known to share needles for steroid injections.

Care for Adolescents

While the cost of providing medical care for adolescents is not much different from the cost of caring for adults, the cost of identifying and caring for adolescents with AIDS requires different techniques which go beyond the direct costs of testing and patient care.

Adolescents who are not in school and who are from "working poor" families are very likely to have inadequate or no insurance. Payment, consent, and confidentiality are common barriers which prevent adolescents from receiving care of any kind, but particularly care related to HIV infection. The Employee Benefit Research Institute reported that in 1985, 20 percent of all children under 18 and 33 percent of all children in families whose income was below the poverty level, were uninsured. The National Center for Health Statistics reported that 15 percent of all 12-17 year-olds had no private or public health insurance or were only covered for part of the year (most likely with a special school insurance).

Adolescents with hemophilia face a double burden. The treatment of the hemophilia alone is very expensive. The annual cost of rh clotting factor concentrates vary from as low as $1,000 for a mild case to $75,000 for a severe case. AIDS is an additional financial catastrophe, observes John Williams, Executive Director of Children's Hospital at Stanford University. One of his patients had medical costs of $244,000 for the last year before he died.

Adolescents, Knowledge, and Behavior

A survey published in the May 1987 issue of Pediatrics revealed that 70 percent of a random sampling of Massachusetts youth aged 16-19 were sexually active, but only 15 percent had changed their sexual behavior because of concern about AIDS; and only 20 percent of those who had changed their behavior used effective methods.

In addition to the sense of invulnerability shared by most adolescents, they still think in "concrete" rather than "abstract" terms. They make decisions based on what they can see, not the long term effects. Peer pressure is at its strongest at this age and often takes precedence over risks. All humans are subject to and tend toward denial, but this age may suffer the most.

Ralph J. DiClemente, et. al., in "Adolescents and AIDS: A Survey of Knowledge, Attitudes and Beliefs about AIDS in San Francisco," (American Journal of Public Health. 1986, Vol. 76, No.12, 1443-1445) investigated 628 students aged 14-18 years; 141 were Hispanic, 226 were black, 261 were white. Slightly more than half were males. While 92 percent understood that AIDS could be transmitted sexually, only 60 percent knew that condom use could lower the risk of infection. Only two-thirds knew that AIDS was spread through sexual contact. This misinformation was especially noticeable among minority youth, which is consistent with the beliefs of minority adults. (See Chapter XIII).

CHAPTER VII

AIDS IN THE WORKPLACE

The nation's leading companies and organizations have made considerable attempts to address the issue of AIDS in the workplace. In October 1987, more than 200 representatives from 73 major companies met at a conference titled, "AIDS: Corporate America Responds," initiated and underwritten by Allstate Insurance Company. The purpose of the conference was to help those in business better understand and cope with the complexities of AIDS. They formed task forces which worked together to prepare position papers on key issues, such as human resource, legal issues, health services, and corporate communications. The conference reconvened in January 1988 to present the task force recommendations. The results of the January meeting were released in AIDS: Corporate America Responds and is available through Allstate Insurance Company, Springbrook, Illinois.

The recommendations include the development of an AIDS policy that, among other things, defines the company position in order to reduce employee fear and uncertainty. Some of the issues the policy should address are commitment to protecting the health of all employees, while providing a safe work environment. At the same time it needs to include the commitment to treat AIDS as any other life-threatening illness, and that those with AIDS who are medically fit and able to perform their duties will be permitted to work. Human resource issues need to be outlined and responsible employees properly trained in dealing the the inevitable problem that will arise. Employee education, which has the primary objective of keeping fear and hysteria to a minimum and preventing the spread of the disease, is strongly advised. The secondary objectives should be to explain and describe what AIDS is, how it is contracted, how it is spread, and what the risks are in the workplace. Employers need to examine what, if any, adjustments to their benefits program will be made to accommodate those with AIDS and plan for current and potential costs.

The answers are not all there, but the fact that many major corporations are asking difficult questions is encouraging. In February 1988, 30 leading employers, including such giants as AT&T, Dow Jones, IBM, Johnson & Johnson, Time, Inc., and Warner-Lambert Company, endorsed a 10-point "bill of rights" on the AIDS issue which had been prepared by the National Leadership Coalition on AIDS. The independent, Washington-based, group was formed by business leaders in 1987 and financed by private foundations to promote corporate action on AIDS. The basic policy says employees with AIDS or those infected by the virus, "are entitled to the same rights and opportunities as people with other serious or life-threatening illnesses." The new code indicates employers should inform workers on AIDS prevention and educate them before a case develops in the workplace. Medical records should be confidential and testing for HIV antibody as a condition of employment should be prohibited.

A SURVEY OF WORKERS

Most of the American public works; most work outside the home; and most work around other people. Perhaps more than any other area of American life (with the exception of schools) the workplace is a true testing ground for people's beliefs and attitudes about AIDS. Dr. David M. Herold of the Center for Work Performance Problems, College of Management of the Georgia Institute of Technology in Atlanta, Georgia, with a grant from the Alcoa Corporation conducted a telephone interview of over 2,000 workers, who were 18 years of age or over, full-time, civilian employees and who were not self-employed. The results of the survey, published in Employees' Reaction to AIDS in the Workplace (Atlanta, GA: February 1988), have a .95 confidence level that should differ no more than +/- 3 percent from other employees in the U.S. work force who have the same characteristics. The survey focused on the nature of fears concerning contact with AIDS patients, willingness to accommodate AIDS workers, issues which effect a worker's attitudes about AIDS, and the extent of personal knowledge of AIDS victims.

Fear About Contact

Two-thirds of those surveyed would be concerned about using the same bathroom as someone who has AIDS, while two out of five would be concerned about eating in the same cafeteria. Dr. Herold points out that this fearfulness could cause potential disruption in the normal activities of an organization. A factor that could directly affect the productivity of a workplace is the reluctance of 37 percent of workers to share tools and equipment with an employee with AIDS. In all instances the fear was inversely proportionate to the educational level of the employee questioned.

Accommodating

In spite of the relatively high level of fear of contact expressed in the previous set of questions, these same workers showed a strong measure of sympathy for those workers who have AIDS. Three-quarters were in favor of making special work accommodations if the AIDS-afflicted co-worker's

"If a person were known to have AIDS":

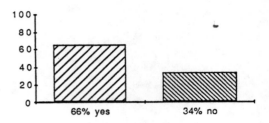

Would you be concerned about using the same bathroom?

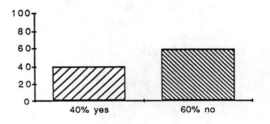

Would you be concerned about eating in the same cafeteria?

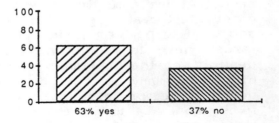

Would you be willing to share tools or equipment with the individual?

% FEARING

Education Level	Sharing Bathroom	Sharing Cafeteria	Sharing Tools
Some High School	72	49	47
High School grads.	74	48	42
College grads.	61	36	33
Advanced degrees	48	25	26

Source: Herold, David M. Employees' Reactions to AIDS in the Workplace. Center on Work Performance Problems, Georgia Institute of Technology, College of Management, Atlanta, GA. 1988

health deteriorated, and over 80 percent offered to provide assistance in helping the worker perform his or her job. These comments almost directly contradicted the fears expressed earlier. How can one "accommodate" and "help" these workers without contact? Dr. Herold suggests that a cynical explanation might be that helping and accommodating translates into making it easier for the AIDS workers to stay off the job, but that more research is needed in this area. Unlike the issue of fear, few differences existed in the sex, race, education, or job type of those who voiced support for special work arrangements or willingness to help.

Issue Affecting Beliefs

More than two out of five workers believed it was likely that people with other illnesses were really covering up the fact that they had AIDS. More than one-third were unsure, and less than one-quarter believed it was unlikely. Dr. Herold points out that problems could develop if workers fear that fellow workers with diseases which have similar symptoms to AIDS (leukemia, skin cancer, and pneumonia) really have AIDS. If the worker falls into a high risk group (e.g., homosexual, suspected IV drug user) the danger of such rumors are even greater.

One possible explanation for the paranoia seen in the original question about contact with AIDS workers, is that a large percentage, more than one-third, do not believe the information given out by the Centers for Disease Control and other government agencies about the transmission of AIDS, i.e, that transmission is only through sexual contact and blood contamination. Those with a high school education or less are less likely to believe the evidence presented about AIDS transmission.

Personal Knowledge

Twice as many people in this select survey reported knowing someone who has AIDS than did in the National Health Interview Survey. (See Chapter XIII) This may be partially explained by the fact that most people who have AIDS are in the age range of people who are still working, so they would

"If a person were known to have AIDS":

Would you favor making special work arrangements for the individual if his or her health deteriorated?

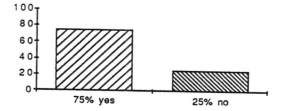

Would you be willing to help the individual perform aspects of the job with which he or she was having difficulty?

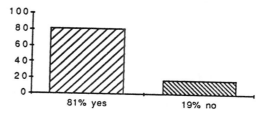

What are the chances that people who are thought to have various illnesses are really covering up the fact that they have AIDS?

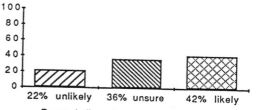

Do you believe the reported evidence that AIDS can only be transmitted by sexual contact or blood contamination?

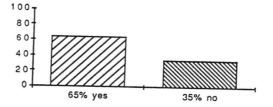

Do you personally know anyone who has the disease AIDS or who has died from it?

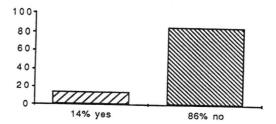

Source: Herold, David M. Employees' Reactions to AIDS in the Workplace. Center on Work Performance Problems, Georgia Institute of Technology, College of Management, Atlanta, GA. 1988

be their peers. These findings show that one out of seven, or 14 percent of those questioned, knew someone who had the disease or who had died from it. As noted earlier, this percentage is expected to increase as many persons who presently have the virus eventually fall victim to the disease. Professional or non-profit employees were more likely to have personal knowledge of an AIDS patient (20 percent and 21 percent, respectively) than blue-collar employees (9 percent). One-fourth of those with advanced degrees knew someone with AIDS, while 9 percent of those with some high school education did.

Concerns and Recommendations

In closing, Dr. Herold points out that workers' attitudes and beliefs about AIDS may soon contribute to significant concerns or problems. Perceptions by management that AIDS is unique and has no affect on their workplace, or that AIDS can be treated like any other disease, and that educating employees about AIDS is a sufficient precaution to ward off fear, may have to be re-examined.

Education about AIDS needs to focus as much on how one does not get AIDS as on how one gets it. Credibility of and often identification with the source as well as level of content are vital to the effectiveness of AIDS education. A message delivered to a union audience would be more readily received if delivered by a fellow union member than by a management team.

Dr. Herold concludes that a multi-faceted corporate response is needed. The medical, legal, and human resources department, as well as union members need to form a task force to examine all aspects of the situation. Outside help might need to be brought in as well. The job of developing an AIDS policy is too great for only one area of the corporation to handle alone.

CHAPTER VIII

THOSE IN SPECIAL SETTINGS

PREVALENCE IN SPECIAL SETTINGS

Persons in certain special circumstances may require special public health procedures to prevent and control of HIV infection. People in such special situations include prisoners, prostitutes, those with tuberculosis, health care workers, and those in the military.

Prisoners

Prisoners present special health concerns due to exposure to drugs and homosexual activity while incarcerated. The National Institute of Justice and the American Correctional Association jointly sponsored AIDS in Correctional Facilities: Issues and Options (WDC, 1987), a study based largely on questionnaires sent to the correctional departments of all 50 states, the federal prison system, and 37 large city and county jails. The initial findings (as of November 1985 –January 1986) resulted from an overwhelming 95 percent response rate – 100 percent for the state and federal system; and 89 percent for city-county systems.

Twenty-five state and federal correctional systems reported 455 confirmed AIDS case, while 20 large city and county systems reported 311 cases of AIDS among inmates, for a total of 766 correctional AIDS cases. These were cumulative cases counting all cases since the systems began keeping records.

By the time the survey was released in October 1986, the number had risen to 1,232 confirmed AIDS cases among inmates in 58 responding federal, state, and local correctional systems. Thirty-one federal and state systems reported 784 cases, up 72 percent from 1985, while 27 city and county jail systems reported 448 cases, up 44 percent from the previous year. In just a short period, AIDS cases among all systems had increased 61 percent, although this was less than the national increase of 79 percent from 14,519 cases to 26,002 cases during the same time period. As with the original study, these figures are cumulative, counting all cases reported since the record-keeping began.

Twenty-three state and federal systems reported 174 current cases, while six city/county systems reported 29. State and federal officials reported that 463 inmates had died from AIDS while in prison; while the city/county systems reported 66 inmate deaths. Almost half, or 254 of the deaths, had occurred since the original survey.

The distribution of AIDS cases in the correctional systems was quite uneven. While 10 more systems than the previous year reported at least one case,

DISTRIBUTION OF CONFIRMED AIDS CASES AMONG INMATES, BY TYPE OF SYSTEM

Range of Total AIDS Cases	State/Federal Prison Systems							
	Original Survey: November 1985				Update Survey: October 1986			
	n systems	%	n cases	%	n systems	%	n cases	%
0	26	51%	0	0%	20	39%	0	0%
1-3	15	29	24	5	15	29	22	3
4-10	5	10	30	7	9	18	56	7
11-25	2	4	42	9	1	2	23	3
26-50	1	2	33	7	3	6	101	13
51-100	1	2	95	21	1	2	57	7
>100	1	2	231	51	2	4	525	67
Total	51	100%	455	100%	51	100%	784	100%

Range of Total AIDS Cases	City/County Jail Systems							
	Original Survey: November 1985				Update Survey: October 1986			
	n systems	%	n cases	%	n systems	%	n cases	%
0	13	39%	0	0%	6	18%	0	0%
1-3	10	30	16	5	12	36	24	5
4-10	7	21	43	14	10[a]	30	60	13
11-25	1	3	12	4	3	9	39	9
26-50	1	3	40	13	1	3	40	9
51-100	0	0	0	0	0	0	0	0
>100	1	3	200	64	1	3	285	64
Total	33	99%[b]	311	100%	33	99%[b]	448	100%

Source: NIJ/ACA Questionnaire Responses.

[a] Two systems in this category at the time of the original study failed to respond to the 1986 survey. Therefore, the numbers reported are from the 1985 survey.

[b] Due to rounding.

REGIONAL DISTRIBUTION OF TOTAL AIDS CASES BY TYPE OF SYSTEM
(Federal Bureau of Prisons Excluded)

Region	State Prison Systems			
	Original Survey: November 1985		Update Survey: October 1986	
	n Cases	% of Total	n Cases	% of Total
New England[a]	16	3.7%	34	4.6%
Mid-Atlantic[b]	327	75.5	531	71.3
E.N. Central[c]	6	1.4	19	2.6
W.N. Central[d]	0	0.0	1	0.1
S. Atlantic[e]	49	11.3	88	11.8
E.S. Central[f]	1	0.2	5	0.7
W.S. Central[g]	12	2.8	28	3.8
Mountain[h]	2	0.5	2	0.3
Pacific[i]	20	4.6	37	5.0
Total	433	100.0%	745	100.2%[k]

Region	City/County Jail Systems			
	Original Survey: November 1985		Update Survey: October 1986	
	n Cases	% of Total	n Cases	% of Total
New England[a]	0	0.0%	0	0.0%
Mid-Atlantic[b]	222	71.4	307[j]	68.5
E.N. Central[c]	8	2.6	17	3.8
W.N. Central[d]	1	0.3	2	0.4
S. Atlantic[e]	24	7.7	27[j]	6.0
E.S. Central[f]	0	0.0	0	0.0
W.S. Central[g]	3	1.0	6	1.3
Mountain[h]	1	0.3	6	1.3
Pacific[i]	52	16.7	83	18.5
Total	311	100.0%	448	99.8%[k]

[a] Maine, New Hampshire, Vermont, Massachusetts, Rhode Island, Connecticut

[b] New York, New Jersey, Pennsylvania

[c] Ohio, Indiana, Illinois, Michigan, Wisconsin

[d] Minnesota, Iowa, Missouri, North Dakota, South Dakota, Nebraska, Kansas

[e] Delaware, Maryland, District of Columbia, Virginia, West Virginia, North Carolina, South Carolina, Georgia, Florida

[f] Kentucky, Tennessee, Alabama, Mississippi

[g] Arkansas, Louisiana, Oklahoma, Texas

[h] Montana, Idaho, Wyoming, Colorado, New Mexico, Arizona, Utah, Nevada

[i] Washington, Oregon, California, Alaska, Hawaii

[j] One system in this region failed to submit a follow-up questionnaire. We used the numbers reported on the original questionnaire.

[k] Due to rounding

Source: AIDS in Correctional Facilities: Issues and Options, National Institute of Justice, (WDC, 1987)

the majority still had fewer than four cases. On the other hand, three state and federal systems and one responding city/-county system had more than 50 cases. Three state systems, (New York, New Jersey, Pennsylvania) accounted for 74 percent of the cumulative total AIDS cases.

A New York Profile

Acquired Immune Deficiency Syndrome: A Demographic Profile of New York State Inmate Mortalities 1981-1986 (Albany, NY, September 1987 Update), a study of 177 inmate deaths from AIDS prepared by the New York State Commission of Corrections, reported that almost all (96 percent) were males, and three-fourths were between 25 and 29 years old. Over 90 percent were admitted IV drug abusers, 45 percent were Hispanic, 43 percent were black, and 86 percent came from New York City.

As of December 1987, the New York State prisons system had counted 597 AIDS cases since 1981. Of these, 346 has died, 152 had left the system, and the remaining 99 were still incarcerated. The report found that New York State prisoners with AIDS lived only half as long as those with AIDS who were not in prison. One likely explanation may be that medical care in prison is not equal to medical care outside. With over one-third of all AIDS cases in the U.S. coming from New York, it is not surprising that the state's correctional system has been overloaded. The report notes that 57 percent of the deaths were of persons who had been in the correctional system for 1-18 months; 27 percent for 19-36 months; 12 percent for 37-54 months; and 3 percent for 4 1/2 to six years. Two inmates had been in prison 6 1/2 to seven years when they died.

Alvin J. Bronstein, Executive Director of the National Prison Project of the American Civil Liberties Union (ACLU), testified before the House Judiciary Committee's Subcommittee on Courts, Civil Liberties and the Administration of Justice that medical care for prisoners with AIDS was a particularly serious problem. Of particular importance was the refusal of some prison health officials to treat certain ailments. Another problem was the placement of prisoners with AIDS in wards or rooms with persons with infectious diseases. Because of the weakening of the immune system, AIDS victims are far more vulnerable to other diseases and opportunistic infections than other patients. Prisoners are also less likely to receive the latest treatment and to be treated with the expensive drug AZT, the medication found to prolong life for some AIDS patients.

Prostitutes

Women who exchange sex for money or drugs are at particular risk for HIV infection. In order to determine the prevalence and risk factors for HIV infection in U.S. prostitutes, the CDC collaborates with several other agencies in an ongoing, study of prostitutes in seven areas - Atlanta (GA), Colorado Springs (CO), Las Vegas (NV), Los Angeles (CA), Miami (FL), Newark-Jersey City-Paterson (NJ), and San Francisco (CA). Some agencies draw test results from imprisoned women, others rely on medical situations such as sexually transmitted disease (STD) clinics; still others place ads in newspapers, pass out pamphlets, or make direct contact in the street. Because of the many different information-gathering methods, these findings may not be representative of all female prostitutes in these areas.

The CDC, in "Antibody to human immunodeficiency virus female prostitutes," (Morbidity and Mortality Weekly Report (MMWR), March 27, 1987) reported that the prevalence of AIDS in prostitutes was similar to that of other women in the seven research areas. The prevalence of HIV antibody was greatest in northern New Jersey and Miami. In southern Nevada, where only one woman had been reported with AIDS by March 1987, none of the 34 prostitutes tested positive. (Nevada, incidentally, is the only state with legalized prostitution in certain counties. Because prostitution is legal there, as in many European countries, health officials strictly regulate the business. In addition, the prostitutes may likely be more careful in how they practice their business.)

In all seven areas, black and Hispanic women showed higher rates of AIDS than white women. The incidence of AIDS was 359.6 per 1 million black women; 40.2 per million Hispanic women; 25.3 per 1 million white women; and 16.2 per million among other (Asian and Native American) women. Similarly, black and Hispanic prostitutes had a higher prevalence of HIV antibody (15 percent) than white or other prostitutes (7 percent).

Drug use among prostitutes is very common and is associated with HIV infection and AIDS in women regardless of ethnic or racial background. Half of those interviewed had histories of IV drug abuse, and 47 of 62 prostitutes (76 percent) with the HIV antibody had injected drugs.

Four out of five of the prostitutes indicated that at least one of their partners had used a condom, a measure recognized as a preventative if properly used. The husbands and boyfriends of these women were less likely to have used a condom during vaginal contact than were the clients (16 percent vs. 78 percent). Fewer than 5 percent of the prostitutes reported condom use with each vaginal exposure during the last five years. Eleven percent of the 546 prostitutes who were unprotected during vaginal contact tested positive for HIV antibody. None of the 22 who reported their partners always used condoms tested positive.

Tuberculosis Patients

HIV antibody in female prostitutes and reported AIDS cases in women — selected cities, United States, March 10, 1987

	Female prostitutes		Women with AIDS[*]	
	HIV-antibody positive/tested	Percent positive	No.	Cases/ 1,000,000[†]
Eastern United States				
Atlanta	1/92	(1.1)	8	12.5
Miami	47/252	(18.7)	100	145.3
Newark-Jersey City-Paterson	32/56	(57.1)	143	526.2
Western United States				
Colorado Springs	1/71	(1.4)	1	9.6
Las Vegas	0/34	(0.0)	1	16.0
Los Angeles	8/184	(4.3)	26	21.7
San Francisco	9/146	(6.2)	21	71.9

[*]Includes 45 women (≥16 years of age) from Miami and one from Newark who were born in countries where heterosexual transmission is believed to play a major role.
[†]Rate based on the number of females (≥16 years of age) reported as residing in the urban area or place of study (26).

TABLE 2. Risk factors for HIV antibody in female prostitutes and for AIDS in women, by race or ethnic group — selected cities, United States, March 10, 1987

	Female prostitutes[*]		Women with AIDS[†]	
	HIV-antibody positive/tested	Percent positive	No.	Percent of total
Black or Hispanic				
IV-drug abuser	31/124	(25.0)	108	(43.0)
Other, unknown	12/156[§]	(7.7)	143	(57.0)
Total	43/280	(15.4)	251	(100.0)
White or other				
IV-drug abuser	16/157	(10.2)	26	(53.1)
Other, unknown	3/127[¶]	(2.4)	23	(46.9)
Total	19/284	(6.7)	49	(100.0)

[*]Analysis restricted to the 564 study participants (of 835 tested) who answered the question regarding IV-drug abuse.
[†]Includes 46 women who were born in countries where heterosexual transmission is believed to play a major role, who were reported to CDC as meeting the surveillance case definition for AIDS, and who were residents of one of the seven research sites.
[§]Odds ratio = 4.0; 95% confidence interval = 2.0-8.2.
[¶]Odds ratio = 4.7; 95% confidence interval = 1.3-16.5.

Source: Report on AIDS, June 1986-May 1987, Centers for Disease Control, (WDC, 1987)

Clinical tuberculosis (TB) is a possible opportunistic disease which can occur in an immune system infected with HIV. For the first time in recent memory, the incidence has risen, particularly in areas where HIV infection has reached high levels.

Florida

In 1985, tuberculosis cases increased 7 percent over the previous year in Florida. Concern about a possible association between HIV and increased tuberculosis occurrence led some researchers to evaluate data on both AIDS and TB. Subgroups were identified and their characteristics compared. The subgroups were: AIDS patients with or without tuberculosis (AID/TB and AIDS/non-TB); and tuberculosis patients with and without AIDS (TB/AIDS and TB/non-AIDS).

Of the nearly 1,100 persons meeting the CDC surveillance definition for AIDS in Florida between 1981 and 1985, 109 (10 percent) were also diagnosed between 1978 and 1985 as having had TB. From 1981 to 1984, the number of persons diagnosed each year as having had AIDS, who also had TB, rose from zero to 55. The following year, 1985, the number dropped to 26. The length of time between the report of tuberculosis and AIDS diagnosis ranged from seven years before to 15 months after AIDS was diagnosed. The median interval was three months before AIDS diagnosis. Patients with both AIDS and TB were overwhelmingly black, male, and born in foreign countries. Interestingly, however, half of those with both diseases were born in countries which were not identified as risk countries for heterosexual transmission, such as Haiti, or countries of central Africa. Less than one-quarter of AIDS/TB victims were reported as homosexual or bisexual men.

Of the 7,241 cases of tuberculosis reported in Florida between 1981-1985, 105 (2 percent) also were AIDS cases. (This number is four fewer than the number mentioned in the preceding paragraph because they had been reported before 1981, when no detailed information on the cases was available. They were subsequently dropped from the analysis). The number and proportion generally rose over this time period. Of the 105 TB/AIDS patients, 65 (60 percent) were reported to also have had TB while residing in Dade County (Miami) and 23 (22 percent) were living in Palm Beach County. When TB/AIDS patients were compared with TB/non-AIDS patients, the TB/AIDS patients tended to be younger (median age 30 versus 40) and were more frequently black (79 percent versus 51 percent), male (83 percent versus 71 percent), and foreign born (60 percent versus 21 percent).

Characteristics of acquired immunodeficiency syndrome (AIDS) cases with and without tuberculosis (TB)—Florida, 1981-1985*

Characteristic	AIDS/TB (n = 109) No. (%)		AIDS/non-TB (n = 985) No. (%)		Statistical significance
Age					
Median	30		34		
Mean	33.6		34.6		Not significant
Race/ethnicity					
Black	88	(80.7)	363	(36.9)	
White	12	(11.0)	495	(50.3)	p < 0.001
Hispanic	9	(8.3)	122	(12.4)	
Other	0	(0.0)	5	(0.5)	
Sex					
Female	18	(16.5)	110	(11.2)	
Male	91	(83.5)	875	(88.8)	Not significant
Country of origin					
U.S.	44	(40.4)	737	(74.8)	
Foreign	65	(59.6)	248	(25.2)	p < 0.001
AIDS risk factors					
Homosexual/ bisexual men	23	(21.1)	609	(61.8)	
IV drug abuse	20	(18.3)	128	(13.0)	p < 0.001
Born NIR ctry[†]	55	(50.5)	127	(12.9)	
Other/none	11	(10.1)	121	(12.3)	

*Because only aggregate data were available for certain characteristics, no adjustments were made in the analysis.

[†]No identified risk country—country in which heterosexual transmission of human T-lymphotropic virus type III/lymphadenopathy-associated virus is thought to play a major role.

Characteristics of tuberculosis (TB) cases with and without acquired immunodeficiency syndrome (AIDS)—Florida, 1981-1985

Characteristic	TB/AIDS (n = 105) No. (%)		TB/non-AIDS (n = 7,136) No. (%)		Statistical significance
Age					
Median	30		49		p < 0.001
Mean	33.2		48.7		
Race					
Black	83	(79.0)	3,613	(50.5)	
White	22	(21.0)	3,380	(47.4)	p < 0.001
Other	0	(0.0)	143	(2.0)	
Ethnicity					
Hispanic	11	(10.5)	685	(9.6)	
Non-Hispanic	94	(89.5)	6,451	(90.4)	Not significant
Sex					
Female	18	(17.1)	2,084	(29.2)	
Male	87	(82.9)	5,052	(70.8)	0.001 < p < 0.01
Country of origin					
U.S.	42	(40.0)	5,610	(78.6)	
Foreign	63	(60.0)	1,526	(21.4)	p < 0.001
Form of TB					
Pulmonary	65	(61.9)	6,331	(88.7)	
Pleural	1	(0.1)	216	(3.0)	
Lymphatic	20	(19.0)	167	(2.3)	p < 0.001
Miliary	10	(9.5)	96	(1.3)	
Other	9	(8.6)	326	(4.6)	

Source: Report on AIDS, June 1986–May 1987, Centers for Disease Control, (WDC, 1987)

Back in 1985, those who researched the Florida data believed that the 10 percent overlap of TB and AIDS patients suggested an association between the two diseases. Those AIDS patients who had TB may have had latent (present, but inactive) tuberculosis infection for years, which progressed to clinical (active) TB as a result of the immunodeficiency caused by the AIDS virus. Because radiology cannot distinguish between the TB in AIDS patients from the primary forms found in patients without AIDS, it cannot be certain that the tuberculosis infection is not a new one.

New York

The CDC, in "Tuberculosis and Acquired Immundeficiency Syndrome – New York City," (Morbidity and Mortality Weekly Report, December 11, 1987) reported that TB cases in New York City (NYC) had increased substantially in recent years, largely due to coexisting HIV and Mycobacterium tuberculosis infection.

Intravenous (IV) drug abuse and homosexuality/bisexuality among adult and adolescent AIDS patients* with TB (TB/AIDS) and without TB, by race/ethnicity and AIDS risk factor — New York City, 1981-1985

	IV Drug Abuse			Homo/Bisexuality			Both Factors			Neither Factor		
		TB/AIDS Cases			TB/AIDS Cases			TB/AIDS Cases			TB/AIDS Cases	
Race/Ethnicity	AIDS Cases	No.	(%)	AIDS Cases	No.	(%)	AIDS Cases	No.	(%)	AIDS Cases	No.	(%)
Black, Non-Haitian	669	70	(10)	509	21	(4)	101	12	(12)	107	4	(4)
White, Non-Hispanic	191	9	(5)	1,803	36	(2)	107	4	(4)	61	0	(0)
Hispanic	555	44	(8)	436	23	(5)	74	6	(8)	88	3	(3)
Total	1,415	123	(9)	2,748	80	(3)	282	22	(8)	256	7	(3)

*Excludes 148 Haitian AIDS patients, 29 of whom also had TB, and 43 patients with other or unknown race/ethnicity, none of whom also had TB.

Reported tuberculosis cases, by year — New York City, 1981-1986

Adult and adolescent TB patients with AIDS (TB/AIDS) and without AIDS, by demographic group and clinical characteristics of TB — New York City, 1979-1985

	TB/AIDS (n = 261)		TB Only (n = 10,970)	
Characteristics at TB Diagnosis	No.	(%)	No.	(%)
Sex				
Male	226	(87)	7,351	(67)
Female	35	(13)	3,619	(33)
Age 20-49 Years				
Yes	244	(93)	6,219	(57)
No	17	(7)	4,751	(43)
Disease Sites				
Multiple*	62	(24)	415	(4)
One, Extrapulmonary	58	(22)	1,741	(16)
One, Pulmonary	141	(54)	8,814	(80)
Tuberculin Skin Test†				
Nonreactive	50	(58)	792	(18)
Reactive	36	(42)	3,686	(82)
Chest X-ray§				
Normal	13	(8)	269	(3)
Abnormal, Noncavitary	131	(80)	5,410	(66)
Abnormal, Cavitary	20	(12)	2,576	(31)

Adult and adolescent AIDS patients with TB (TB/AIDS) and without TB, by race/ethnicity and AIDS risk factor — New York City, 1981-1985

	TB/AIDS (n=261)		AIDS Only (n=4,631)	
Characteristics	No.	(%)	No.	(%)
Race/Ethnicity				
Black, Non-Haitian	107	(41)	1,279	(28)
Haitian	29	(11)	119	(3)
Hispanic	76	(29)	1,077	(23)
White, Non-Hispanic	49	(19)	2,113	(46)
Other/Unknown	0	–	43	(1)
Risk Factor				
IV Drug Abuse	127	(49)	1,303	(28)
Homosexuality/Bisexuality	81	(31)	2,709	(58)
Both of Above	22	(8)	265	(6)
Other	31	(12)	354	(8)

*Includes at least one extrapulmonary site.
†Includes only patients with known tuberculin skin test results.
§Includes only those with pulmonary disease and known chest X-ray results.

Source: "Tuberculosis and Acquired Immunodeficiency Syndrome - New York City," Morbidity and Mortality Weekly Report, December 11, 1987

60

Between 1985 and 1986, TB cases increased by 593 cases (from 1,1630 to 2,223 cases - 36 percent). This increase was greater than that for any state or other city in the nation. Recorded cases nationwide increased only 2 percent.

New York City and State officials conducted a special study to determine whether the increase of TB cases might by related to AIDS, especially in light of the fact that the increased TB incidence was among males 20-49 years of age, the group accounting fro 80 percent of all New York City AIDS patients. Using the same categories as the Florida study, the researchers compared the TB registry for 1979 through 1985 and the AIDS registry for 1981.

The researchers found 261 patients common to both registries (TB/AIDS). These AIDS victims made up 2 percent of the 11,231 adult and adolescent TB patients from 1979-1985 and 5 percent of the 4,892 adult and adolescent AIDS patients from 1981-1985. The overwhelming majority were males (87 percent); 52 percent were black; 29 percent, Hispanic; and 19 percent, white. The median age for TB/AIDS patients was 34 years. A majority (65 percent) were diagnosed with TB within 6 months before or after being diagnosed with AIDS.

TB/AIDS patients were similar to TB patients without AIDS in median age (34 years compared to 36 years) and gender. However, TB/AIDS patients were more likely to be black (non-Haitian as well as Haitian), and Hispanic than AIDS patients without TB. Moreover, TB/AIDS patients reported IV drug use more frequently and homosexual/bisexual activity less frequently than patients with AIDS alone. The data, illustrated in the accompanying tables, when adjusted for race/ethnicity, shows that those AIDS patients who were IV drug abusers were significantly more likely to develop TB than those who were not. TB/AIDS patients were younger (median age at TB diagnosis was 34 years compared with 44 years) and more likely to be male than those patients with TB and not AIDS.

CDC researchers believe that data from this and other studies suggest that HIV is causing a resurgence of TB in New York City. The increase in TB cases concentrated in the sex and age groups of the majority of NYC AIDS cases - the relatively high proportion of AIDS cases who also have clinically active TB (5 percent); and the proximity in time of AIDS and TB diagnoses among those who have both diseases support the theory of association.

The results of a study presented at the Third International Conference on AIDS, Washington, D.C. June 1-5, 1987, "Evidence for a casual association between HIV infection and increasing tuberculosis incidence in NYC," by R.L. Stoneburner, et al, probably presents the strongest evidence to date on the association. A cohort of 519 IV drug users in New York City followed from 1984 through 1986 produced 279 persons who showed evidence of HIV infection or clinical AIDS. Of these, 12 developed TB. On the other hand, none of the remaining 240 HIV-negative persons developed TB.

HEALTH CARE WORKERS WITH AIDS

Occupational information was available for 46,532 of the 55,315 adults with AIDS on March 14, 1988. Just over 5 percent (2,586) were classified as health-care workers. A corresponding proportion of the U.S. labor force, (5.7 percent) was employed in health services.

The District of Columbia, Puerto Rico, and all but four states have reported health-care workers with AIDS. As with other AIDS patients, the median was 35 years; males accounted for 91.6 percent of health-care workers with AIDS and 92.4 percent of other patients with AIDS. The majority of health-care workers with AIDS (62.8 percent) and of other AIDS patients (60.5 percent) were white.

Almost all (95 percent) of the health-care workers with AIDS were in known transmission categories, but less likely than other persons with AIDS to be IV drug users and more likely to be homosexual or bisexual men. They were also less likely than other persons with AIDS to have a known risk factor. In other words, far more of them than of the general population reported having no identified risk, no reason for having become infected. As of March 14, 1988, state and local health departments had completed investigations for 121 of the 215 health-care workers who were initially reported with an undetermined risk factor. Risk factors were found for 80 of them (66 percent). Of the remainder for whom a risk factor could not be identified, 41 (30.4 percent) could not be reclassified after follow-up; 20 (14.8 percent) had either died or refused to be interviewed; and 74 (65.8 percent) are still under investigation.

Generally, 5.3 percent of health-care workers with AIDS have an undetermined risk, in other words, those with the disease who do not fall into any known risk category. The proportion of such health-care workers has increased from 1.5 percent in 1982 to 6.2 percent in 1987, while there have been similar increases among other AIDS patients. Previous experience suggests that other risk factors for HIV infection will be identified when further investigations are completed. One out of 10 of all reported AIDS patients with undetermined risk are health-care workers.

Comparison of health-care workers with AIDS and other AIDS patients reported to CDC, by transmission category — through March 14, 1988

Transmission Category	Health-Care Workers with AIDS		Other AIDS Patients	
	No.	(%)	No.	(%)
Homosexual or Bisexual Male	1,916	(74.1)*	28,820	(64.1)
Heterosexual Intravenous Drug Abuser	161	(6.2)*	8,263	(18.4)
Homosexual or Bisexual Male and Intravenous Drug Abuser	187	(7.2)	3,267	(7.3)
Hemophilia/Coagulation Disorder	20	(0.8)	451	(1.0)
Heterosexual	119	(4.6)	1,772	(3.9)
Blood/Blood Component Recipient	47	(1.8)	1,105	(2.5)
Other[†]	1	(<1.0)	0	(0.0)
Undetermined[§]	135	(5.3)*	1,268	(2.8)
Total	2,586	(100.0)	44,946	(100.0)

*p<0.001, chi square analysis.
[†]Represents health-care worker who seroconverted to HIV and developed AIDS after documented needlestick exposure to blood.
[§]Includes patients who are under investigation, who died or refused interview, or for whom no risk was identified after follow-up.

HIV infection among health-care workers, by type of exposure and body fluid — CDC Prospective Study, August 15, 1983–December 31, 1987

Type of Exposure	No. of Health-Care Workers with Exposure to				No. of Infections
	Blood	Saliva	Urine	Other/Unknown	
Parenteral (needle-stick or cut with sharp object)	870	7	3	21	4*
Contamination of mucous-membrane, open wound, or nonintact skin	104	42	12	11	0

*All four health-care workers had parenteral exposure to HIV-infected blood; risk is 4/870, or 0.5% (upper bound of 95% confidence interval = 1.1%).

HIV-infected health-care workers with no reported nonoccupational risk factors and for whom case histories have been published in the scientific literature

Cases with Documented Seroconversion

Case	Occupation	Country	Type of Exposure	Source	Reference
1*	NS[†]	United States	Needlestick	AIDS patient	This report
2	NS	United States	Needlestick	AIDS patient	(4,6)
3	NS	United States	Needlestick	AIDS patient	(5)
4	NS	United States	2 Needlesticks	AIDS patient, HIV-infected patient	(5)
5	NS	United States	Needlestick	AIDS patient	(9)
6	Nurse	England	Needlestick	AIDS patient	(12)
7	Nurse	France	Needlestick	HIV-infected patient	(13)
8	Nurse	Martinique	Needlestick	AIDS patient	(14)
9	Research lab worker	United States	Cut with sharp object	Concentrated virus	(15,16)
10	Home health-care provider	United States	Cutaneous[§]	AIDS patient	(17)
11	NS	United States	Nonintact skin	AIDS patient	(18)
12	Phlebotomist	United States	Mucous-membrane	HIV-infected patient	(18)
13	Technologist	United States	Nonintact skin	HIV-infected patient	(18)
14	NS	United States	Needlestick	AIDS patient	(19)
15	Nurse	Italy	Mucous-membrane	HIV-infected patient	(20)

Cases without Documented Seroconversion

Case	Occupation	Country	Type of Exposure	Source	Reference
1	NS	United States	Puncture wound	AIDS patient	(3,4)
2	NS	United States	2 Needlesticks	2 AIDS patients	(3)
3	Research lab worker	United States	Nonintact skin	Concentrated virus	(15,16)
4	Home health-care provider	England	Nonintact skin	AIDS patient	(21)
5	Dentist	United States	Multiple needlesticks	Unknown	(22)
6*	Technician	Mexico	Multiple needlesticks and mucous-membrane	Unknown	(23)
7	Lab worker	United States	Needlestick, puncture wound	Unknown	(3)

*Health-care worker diagnosed with AIDS.
[†]NS = not specified.
[§]Mother who provided nursing care for her child with HIV infection; extensive contact with the child's blood and body secretions and excretions occurred; the mother did not wear gloves and often did not wash her hands immediately after exposure.

Source: "Update: Acquired Immunodeficiency Syndrome and Human Immunodeficiency Virus Infection Among Health-Care Workers," Mortality and Morbity Weekly Report, April 22, 1988

One of the 80 for whom a risk factor was identified was a worker who developed AIDS after a well-documented occupational exposure to blood and HIV seroconversion. The worker was accidentally self-injected with several milliliters of blood from a hospitalized AIDS patient while filling a vacuum collection tube. No other risk factor was found for the health-care worker.

Of the 41 who could not be reclassified into a known risk factor after investigation, eight were physicians, four of whom were surgeons; five nurses, eleven nursing assistants or orderlies; seven housekeeping or maintenance workers; four clinical laboratory technicians; one respiratory therapist; one paramedic; one mortician; and two others with no patient or clinical specimen contact. Maintenance workers were the only occupational group significantly more likely to have an undetermined risk.

Seventeen of the 41 with undetermined risk (including 2 of the 7 maintenance workers) reported needlestick and/or mucous membrane exposure to the blood or body fluids of patients during the 10 years prior to their AIDS diagnosis. However, none was known to be HIV infected at the time of exposure nor were they tested at the time of exposure for HIV antibody. None of the remaining workers reported needlesticks or other exposures to blood or bodily fluids.

Others with HIV Infection

By the end of 1987, 1,176 health-care workers were enrolled and tested for HIV antibody in a continuous CDC surveillance of those exposed to blood or other bodily fluids from HIV-infected patients. Of these, 870 had parenteral exposures (needlestick or cut with a sharp object) to blood; 104 had exposure to mucous membranes, an open wound, or nonintact skin. Four of the 870 with parenteral exposure were seropositive for HIV infection. One of these four was not tested until 10 months after the exposure, and also had an HIV-seropositive sexual partner, so a sexually-acquired infection could not be ruled out.

An April 1987 National Institutes of Health study of 103 health-care workers with documented needlestick injuries and 691 health-care workers with more than 2,000 skin or mucous-membrane exposures to blood or other bodily fluids of HIV-infected patients, found none had seroconverted to HIV infection. As of March 15, 1988, a similar study of 235 health-care workers at the University of California with 644 documented needlestick injuries or mucous-membrane exposures had identified one-seroconversion following a needlestick, according to unpublished study data. In addition to these studies, six persons from the U.S. and four persons from other countries who have denied other HIV-infection risk factors have reported seroconverted to HIV after contact.

The CDC cautions that the increasing number of persons being treated for HIV-associated illnesses makes it quite likely that more health care workers will encounter HIV-infected patients. The risk is minimized if workers rigorously follow CDC regulations and use widely-accepted precautions when caring for all patients.

AIDS IN THE MILITARY

In October 1986, the U.S. Department of Defense (DOD) began the controversial policy of screening all applicants for HIV. Large-scale screening of active-duty personnel already had begun in January 1986. The most recent DOD policy, released in April 1987, makes anyone who tests positive for HIV infection not eligible for enlistment or appointment to the military.

The DOD has reported 274 cases of AIDS occurred between 1982 and 1986 among active duty military personnel (1982 - 1; 1983 - 17; 1984 - 28; 1985 - 70; 1986 -158). The full active duty testing in 1987 found that 1.5 per 1,000 active duty personnel were identified as being HIV positive. The rates per 1,000 for each service were: Army, 1.4; Navy, 2.5; Marine Corps, 1.0; and Air Force, 1.0. Those who test positive may have been infected before they entered the service (before screening of applicants was implemented), or may have become infected while in the service.

Policies

All applicants for military service are screened. Those who test positive to two ELISA tests and the Western blot test are not eligible for appointment or enlistment. For those who enter the service through Officers Candidates School or Officers Training School, positive testing results in an honorable or entry level discharge. Those attending service academies, (such as West Point or Annapolis) are asked to leave the academy and are discharged.

Testing over 2 million personnel on active duty is an awesome task, so priorities have been established to test those of greatest concern. The top priority goes to those service personnel in or subject to be sent to areas in the world which have a high risk of endemic disease or with limited medical capabilities; second, those in or with pending assignments to other duty stations overseas; third, those subject to being sent overseas; and fourth, those such as medical personnel involved in caring for HIV-infected patients.

Positive HIV infection is not to be used as a basis for disciplinary action. Once a positive HIV infection has been diagnosed, appropriate civilian and military authorities are notified. Health officials are to initiate preventive measures such as counseling, immediate health care, and counseling of others at risk (including sexual partners, blood banks, and others). Any military personnel, known to be HIV positive, who does not notify sexual partners of his infection, is subject to discharge and disciplinary action.

Active duty personnel found to be have an HIV infection and who are otherwise fit for duty may continue to serve in accordance with military medical standards. Those infected are treated as any other service personnel with progressive illnesses, such as cancer in remission. If there is no physical or neurological impairment, DOD policy states that personnel will not be separated solely on the basis of the HIV infection. However, those who are HIV-infected and are medically determined to be unfit for further duty, will be retired or separated. Infected personnel may request separation as well.

DOD policy limits the use of information obtained from a service member during a confidential epidemiologic assessment interview when the interview is used to discover the source of the infection. This information cannot be used in "a court martial; nonjudicial punishment; involuntary separation (other than for medical reasons); administrative or punitive reduction in grade; denial of promotion; and unfavorable entry in a personnel record; a bar to reenlistment; and any other action considered by the Secretary concerned to be an adverse personnel action." (David F. Burrelli, Acquired Immune Deficiency Syndrome and Military Manpower Policy, Congressional Research Service, WDC, March 23, 1988).

DOD policy does not forbid the use of this information in actions considered "nonadverse." For example, if the interview reveals that the service member became infected through intravenous drug use, he/she could be denied certain assignments (such as deep-sea diving) or the service could revoke or deny a security clearance. These actions should not be unfavorably entered in the person's personnel record.

CHAPTER IX

AIDS AROUND THE WORLD

The origin of AIDS is murky at best, but a great deal of evidence points to the rural areas of Central Africa. While no evidence is conclusive, those who support the Central Africa theory point to the fact that several other viruses which infect monkeys and humans in Africa are closely related to the HIV. They also rely on well-documented proof of a blood sample infected with the virus in Zaire in 1959. How long the virus had been in Africa or if and when it came from someplace else is also unknown.

In the early years of this decade, physicians in Belgium and France found cases of AIDS among wealthy black Africans who came to Europe for treatment of opportunistic infections. About that same time reports of similar infections began cropping up in the United States. Unlike the African cases, which were heterosexual individuals, AIDS hit the homosexual population of the United States during a period of sexual liberation.

TRACKING SINCE 1981

Dr. Jonathan Mann, director of the Special Programme on AIDS for the World Health Organization (WHO), reports that AIDS has appeared in three-quarters of the world's countries since 1981 when it was first recognized as a disease. The largest numbers are believed to be Africa, although the disease is often unrecognized or unreported there. The U.S., with its vigorous surveillance system, accounts for about one-third of the world's estimated reported total. The disease has made significant inroads into Europe and Latin America, but has barely begun to appear in Asian countries, although this may be due to lack of recognition or underreporting. Nonetheless, experts tend to agree that the virus has only recently entered Asia.

Dr. Mann predicts the global toll will climb swiftly, with 150,000 new cases in 1988 alone, bringing the world total to 300,000. · In spite of the reported total of 98,000, Dr. Mann and WHO estimate that at least 150,000 cases of AIDS have already occurred so far around the world.

WHO estimates that 5 million to 10 million persons are already infected with the AIDS virus. If that estimate is correct, there could be 500,000 to 3 million new AIDS cases over the next five years in people already carrying the virus.

Three broad patterns of infection and disease have emerged around the world. In North America, Europe, Australia and New Zealand, the virus has been

AIDS CASES REPORTED TO WHO BY YEAR AS OF: 31/05/1988

Continent	?	1979	1980	1981	1982	1983	1984	1985	1986	1987	1988	Total
Africa	1	0	0	0	3	14	82	207	2672	8257	294	11530
America	0	14	66	278	1066	3223	6361	11765	18433	24804	5333	71343
Asia	0	0	1	0	1	8	4	30	48	138	24	254
Europe	6	0	3	16	67	215	561	1322	2558	6030	1636	12414
Oceania	0	0	0	0	1	6	45	124	244	372	100	892
Total	7	14	70	294	1138	3466	7053	13448	23955	39601	7387	96433

CUMULATIVE AIDS CASES REPORTED TO WHO BY YEAR AS OF: 31/05/1988

Continent	?	1979	1980	1981	1982	1983	1984	1985	1986	1987	1988	Total
Africa	1	0	0	0	3	17	99	306	2978	11235	11529	11530
Americas	0	14	80	358	1424	4647	11008	22773	41206	66010	71343	71343
Asia	0	0	1	1	2	10	14	44	92	230	254	254
Europe	6	0	3	19	86	301	862	2184	4742	10772	12408	12414
Oceania	0	0	0	0	1	7	52	176	420	792	892	892
Total	7	14	84	378	1516	4982	12035	25483	49438	89039	96426	96433

CASES REPORTED BY CONTINENT AS OF: 31/05/1988

Continent	Number of Cases	Number of Countries or Territories Reporting to WHO	Zero Cases	1 or more cases
Africa	11530	50	7	43
Americas	71343	44	4	40
Asia	254	37	16	21
Europe	12414	30	2	28
Oceania	892	14	10	4
Total	96433	175	39	136

CASES REPORTED BY WHO REGION AS OF: 31/05/1988

WHO Region	Number of Cases	Number of Countries or Territories Reporting to WHO	Zero Cases	1 or more cases
AFRO	11474	44	5	39
AMRO	71343	44	4	40
EMRO	104	20	9	11
EURO	12493	32	2	30
SEARO	24	11	7	4
WPRO	995	24	12	12
Total	96433	175	39	136

Source: "Update: Acquired Immunodeficiency Syndrome, 31 May 1988," World Health Organization

known for several years and infects primarily homosexual men and intravenous drug users. In Africa and Haiti, the virus has also been present for some time, but the primary mode of transmission is through heterosexual intercourse. In some parts of Africa, there is still considerable spreading through contaminated transfusions, since screening donated blood in not universal at this time. In Asia, which is seeing the beginning of the virus, many cases can be traced to previous exposure to contaminated blood products or sexual intercourse with infected foreigners.

SCOPE OF THE PROBLEM

By April 1988, 96,433 cases of AIDS had been reported to the World Health Organization (WHO), of which over 61,000 were in the United States. A total of

175 countries are reporting to WHO with 146 nations reporting one or more AIDS cases. Other countries reporting large numbers of cases include France, Uganda, and Brazil, each with over 2,000 cases. Tanzania, the Federal Republic of (West) Germany, Canada, the United Kingdom, and Italy, have each reported over 1,000 cases. WHO officials estimate that in Africa alone, 50,000 people are already showing symptoms of AIDS in spite of the smaller numbers reported.

This reluctance to accurately report AIDS cases is not new. When AIDS was still in its early stages in the U.S., scientists who needed permission to travel to certain African countries, were told they could come, but could not report cases they found there. Central Africa has been hardest hit by AIDS and is believed to have the largest number of infected persons and deaths, despite the published statistics.

AFRICA

Festered in Africa

A recent study directed by Dr. Nzila Nzilambi of Mama Yemo Hospital in Kinshasa, Zaire was based on blood samples taken in a remote province of Zaire in 1976 before the recognition of AIDS as a disease. Over 650 of the samples were tested for HIV, the AIDS virus. Five of those samples, or eight-tenths of 1 percent, were infected. Researchers returned in 1985, sampled 389 people and found three, also eight-tenths of 1 percent to be infected.

The suggestion is that AIDS has festered at stable levels in rural areas of Africa for some time and that urbanization has helped spread the virus with the help of increased sexual activity and the relaxing of traditional tribal values after arrival in the cities. The prevalence of AIDS in rural areas of Africa has not changed in 10 years, according to Dr. Kevin M. DeCock of the American Centers for Disease Control. On the other hand, cities in Africa have witnessed significant growth in terms of population and AIDS over the same time period.

Spread to West Africa

In 1986, health officials identified carriers of the AIDS virus for the first time in Nigeria, Ivory Coast, Ghana, Senegal, Gambia, and Togo. AIDS had previously been primarily restricted to Central Africa. Authorities blame prostitution, which has become very widespread in modern African cities. Infectious disease authorities predict that, in spite of the realization throughout the region that sex can be deadly, it is unlikely that people will become well-informed in time to change their behavior and head off an epidemic.

The pattern is not unlike that of other infectious diseases. A person is exposed to the disease during foreign travel, then it propagates through prostitutes. Of the eight people who died from AIDS in Gambia in 1986, six were prostitutes who had lived in Zaire, the U.S., and the Federal Republic of (West) Germany, all countries where the virus is more common than in West Africa. The eight AIDS victims in Senegal in 1986 had all traveled or lived overseas.

THE IMPACT

The effect of AIDS on the future of the development and economic growth of Third World countries, especially those in Africa, deeply concern many

Based on reports received through 31/05/1988

African Region

Region	Country	1979-1986 Cases	1987 Cases	1987 Rate(a)	1988 Cases to date	Last Report	Cumulative Cases
AFRO	ALGERIA	3	5	0.0	5	26/03/1988	13
AFRO	ANGOLA	6	0	0.0		26/09/1986	3
AFRO	BENIN	2	0	0.1	0	31/12/1987	3
AFRO	BOTSWANA	7	9	0.7	0	27/01/1988	16
AFRO	BURKINA FASO	0	26	0.3	0	30/06/1987	26
AFRO	BURUNDI	269	652	13.0	39	31/01/1988	960
AFRO	CAMEROON	21	4	0.0	0	05/03/1987	25
AFRO	CAPE VERDE	2	2	0.6	0	30/04/1987	4
AFRO	CENTR.AFR.REP.	254	0	0.0	0	31/10/1986	254
AFRO	CHAD	1	0	0.0	0	13/11/1986	1
AFRO	COMOROS	0	0	0.0	0	13/11/1986	0
AFRO	CONGO	250	1000	47.6	0	09/12/1987	1250
AFRO	COTE D'IVOIRE	118	132	1.2	0	20/11/1987	250
AFRO	ETHIOPIA	0	19	0.0	2	14/03/1988	21
AFRO	GABON	0	18	1.5	0	31/03/1988	18*
AFRO	GAMBIA	13	22	2.7	0	08/03/1988	35
AFRO	GHANA	73	72	0.5	0	25/05/1987	145
AFRO	GUINEA	0	4	0.0	0	12/11/1987	4
AFRO	GUINEA BISSAU	0	16	1.7	0	20/11/1987	16
AFRO	KENYA	109	1388	6.2	0	31/12/1987	1497*
AFRO	LESOTHO	1	1	0.0	0	27/11/1987	2
AFRO	LIBERIA	0	2	0.0	0	11/03/1988	2
AFRO	MADAGASCAR	0	0	0.0	0	25/04/1987	0
AFRO	MALAWI	13	570	7.7	0	31/10/1987	583
AFRO	MALI	6	23	0.2	0	14/01/1988	29
AFRO	MAURITANIA	0	0	0.0	0	13/11/1987	0
AFRO	MAURITIUS	0	1	0.0	0	18/12/1987	1
AFRO	MOZAMBIQUE	1	3	0.0	5	30/04/1988	9*
AFRO	NIGER	0	9	0.1	0	14/10/1987	9
AFRO	NIGERIA	0	9	0.0	2	11/03/1988	11
AFRO	REUNION	1	1	0.1	0	27/02/1988	2
AFRO	RWANDA	705	196	2.8	0	30/11/1987	901
AFRO	SAO TOME/PRINCIPE	0	1	0.0	0	11/02/1988	1
AFRO	SENEGAL	0	66	0.9	0	04/12/1987	66
AFRO	SEYCHELLES	0	0	0.0	0	13/11/1987	0
AFRO	SIERRA LEONE	0	0	0.0	0	03/11/1987	0
AFRO	SOUTH AFRICA @	55	46	0.1	13	08/03/1988	114*
AFRO	SWAZILAND	1	6	0.8	0	01/07/1987	7
AFRO	TANZANIA	699	909	3.8	0	17/10/1987	1608
AFRO	TOGO	0	2	0.0	0	10/12/1987	2
AFRO	UGANDA	118	2251	14.1	0	31/10/1987	2369
AFRO	ZAIRE	0	335	1.0	0	30/06/1987	335
AFRO	ZAMBIA	250	286	4.0	218	28/04/1988	754*
AFRO	ZIMBABWE	0	119	1.2	0	30/04/1988	119*
Total for the Region		2977	8211	1.7	286		11474

American Region

Region	Country	1979-1986 Cases	1987 Cases	1987 Rate(a)	1988 Cases to date	Last Report	Cumulative Cases
AMRO	ANGUILLA	0	0	0.0	0	31/03/1988	0*
AMRO	ANTIGUA	2	1	1.0	0	30/06/1987	3
AMRO	ARGENTINA	69	51	0.1	43	31/03/1988	163*
AMRO	BAHAMAS	85	78	33.9	25	31/03/1988	188*
AMRO	BARBADOS	15	40	13.3	0	31/12/1987	55*
AMRO	BELIZE	1	6	3.0	0	31/12/1987	7*
AMRO	BERMUDA	48	27	33.7	0	30/09/1987	75
AMRO	BOLIVIA	1	3	0.0	2	22/01/1988	6
AMRO	BR. VIRGIN ISLANDS	0	0	0.0	0	31/03/1987	0
AMRO	BRAZIL	1389	1361	0.9	206	02/04/1988	2956*
AMRO	CANADA	1030	513	1.9	232	27/04/1988	1775*
AMRO	CAYMAN ISLANDS	1	2	10.2	0	31/12/1987	3*
AMRO	CHILE	22	34	0.2	13	31/12/1987	69*
AMRO	COLOMBIA	30	144	0.4	0	31/12/1987	174*
AMRO	COSTA RICA	16	27	0.9	0	31/03/1988	43*
AMRO	CUBA	1	26	0.2	0	31/12/1987	27
AMRO	DOMINICA	0	4	4.0	0	31/12/1987	4*
AMRO	DOMINICAN REPUBLIC	96	256	3.9	152	31/03/1988	504*
AMRO	ECUADOR	7	32	0.3	0	31/03/1988	39*
AMRO	EL SALVADOR	6	17	0.3	0	31/03/1988	23*
AMRO	FRENCH GUIANA	58	45	56.2	10	31/12/1987	113*
AMRO	GRENADA	3	5	4.5	0	31/12/1987	8*
AMRO	GUADELOUPE	40	34	10.3	0	31/12/1987	74*
AMRO	GUATEMALA	15	19	0.2	0	31/12/1987	34*
AMRO	GUYANA	0	14	0.6	0	31/12/1987	14*
AMRO	HAITI	811	332	5.0	231	31/03/1988	1374*
AMRO	HONDURAS	13	58	1.2	38	31/03/1988	109*
AMRO	JAMAICA	6	37	1.4	13	31/03/1988	56*
AMRO	MARTINIQUE	16	22	6.6	0	31/12/1987	38*
AMRO	MEXICO	789	499	0.6	14	01/04/1988	1302*
AMRO	MONTSERRAT	0	0	0.0	0	30/09/1987	0
AMRO	NICARAGUA	0	0	0.0	0	31/12/1987	0*
AMRO	PANAMA	12	18	0.7	0	31/12/1987	30*
AMRO	PARAGUAY	1	7	0.2	0	31/12/1987	8*
AMRO	PERU	9	60	0.1	0	30/09/1987	69*
AMRO	ST. CHRISTOPHER	1	0	0.2	0	31/12/1987	1
AMRO	ST. LUCIA	3	7	5.3	0	31/12/1987	10*
AMRO	ST. VINCENT	3	5	5.0	0	31/12/1987	8*
AMRO	SURINAME	2	7	1.7	0	31/12/1987	9*
AMRO	TRINIDAD & TOBAGO	134	93	7.1	0	31/12/1987	227*
AMRO	TURKS & CAICOS	2	3	30.0	0	31/12/1987	5*
AMRO	UNITED STATES AM.**	36392	20840	8.5	4348	31/03/1988	61580*
AMRO	URUGUAY	8	6	0.2	0	31/03/1988	20*
AMRO	VENEZUELA	69	71	0.3	0	31/12/1987	140*
Total for the Region		41206	24804	3.6	5333		71343

(a) Rate: 1987 Reported Cases / 100,000 Population

* Updated report

@ Not an active member of the Region

** After revision, Zimbabwe is now reporting 119 cases.

** Puerto Rico included in USA

Source: "Update: Acquired Immunodeficiency Syndrome, 31 May 1988," World Health Organization

Eastern Mediterranean Region

Region	Country	1979-1986 Cases	1987 Cases	1987 Rate(a)	1988 Cases to date	Last Report	Cumulative Cases
EMRO	AFGHANISTAN	0	0	0.0	0	31/12/1987	0
EMRO	BAHRAIN	0	0	0.0	0	31/12/1987	0
EMRO	CYPRUS	1	2	0.2	0	01/06/1987	3
EMRO	DEMOCRATIC YEMEN	0	0	0.0	0	01/06/1987	0
EMRO	DJIBOUTI	0	0	0.0	0	01/10/1987	0
EMRO	EGYPT	0	1	0.0	4	31/12/1987	5
EMRO	IRAN	0	1	0.0	0	31/01/1988	1
EMRO	IRAQ	0	0	0.0	0	31/12/1987	0
EMRO	JORDAN	0	0	0.0	0	24/12/1987	0
EMRO	KUWAIT	0	3	0.1	0	31/12/1987	3
EMRO	LEBANON	0	5	0.0	0	31/12/1987	5
EMRO	LYBIA	0	0	0.0	0	31/12/1987	0
EMRO	MOROCCO	0	9	0.0	0	31/12/1987	9
EMRO	PAKISTAN	0	1	0.0	0	31/12/1987	1
EMRO	QATAR	0	32	10.0	0	31/12/1987	32
EMRO	SOMALIA	0	0	0.0	0	31/12/1987	0
EMRO	SUDAN	0	19	0.0	4	31/12/1987	23
EMRO	SYRIA	0	3	0.0	0	20/03/1988	3
EMRO	TUNISIA	2	17	0.2	0	30/01/1988	19
EMRO	YEMEN	0	0	0.0	0	31/12/1987	0
	Total for the Region	3	93	0.0	8		104

European Region

Region	Country	1979-1986 Cases	1987 Cases	1987 Rate(a)	1988 Cases to date	Last Report	Cumulative Cases
EURO	ALBANIA	0	0	0.0	0	31/03/1988	0*
EURO	AUSTRIA	54	85	1.1	37	03/05/1988	176*
EURO	BELGIUM	230	85	0.8	25	01/05/1988	340*
EURO	BULGARIA	0	3	0.0	0	06/10/1987	3
EURO	CZECHOSLOVAKIA	6	2	0.0	2	31/12/1987	10*
EURO	DENMARK	141	97	1.8	25	01/05/1988	263*
EURO	FED.REP.GERMANY	980	846	1.3	147	30/04/1988	1973*
EURO	FINLAND	14	10	0.2	3	31/03/1988	27*
EURO	FRANCE	1221	1852	3.3	555	31/03/1988	3628*
EURO	GERMAN DEM.REP.	1	5	0.0	0	31/12/1988	6
EURO	GREECE	35	53	0.5	18	31/03/1988	106*
EURO	HUNGARY	1	7	0.0	4	06/05/1988	12*
EURO	ICELAND	4	1	0.4	0	01/05/1988	5*
EURO	IRELAND	14	19	0.5	4	31/03/1988	37*
EURO	ISRAEL	34	13	0.3	11	31/03/1988	58*
EURO	ITALY	590	888	1.5	387	30/04/1988	1865*
EURO	LUXEMBOURG	6	3	0.7	1	01/05/1988	10*
EURO	MALTA	5	3	0.7	2	22/04/1988	10*
EURO	MONACO	0	1	3.7	0	31/12/1987	1
EURO	NETHERLANDS	236	215	1.4	50	01/05/1988	501*
EURO	NORWAY	35	35	0.8	11	07/04/1988	81*
EURO	POLAND	1	2	0.0	0	06/05/1988	3*
EURO	PORTUGAL	46	44	0.4	35	01/05/1988	125*
EURO	ROMANIA	2	2	0.0	0	12/04/1988	4*
EURO	SAN MARINO	0	0	0.0	0	18/02/1988	0*
EURO	SPAIN	264	862	2.2	0	01/04/1988	1126*
EURO	SWEDEN	90	73	0.8	29	30/04/1988	192*
EURO	SWITZERLAND	192	163	2.4	84	31/03/1988	439*
EURO	TURKEY	9	12	0.0	0	31/12/1987	21
EURO	UNITED KINGDOM	571	653	1.1	205	31/03/1988	1429
EURO	USSR	1	3	0.0	0	31/12/1987	4*
EURO	YUGOSLAVIA	8	18	0.0	12	31/03/1988	38*

South East Asia Region

Region	Country	1979-1986 Cases	1987 Cases	1987 Rate(a)	1988 Cases to date	Last Report	Cumulative Cases
SEARO	BANGLADESH	0	0	0.0	0	14/04/1987	0
SEARO	BHUTAN	0	0	0.0	0	14/04/1987	0
SEARO	BURMA	0	0	0.0	0	14/04/1987	0
SEARO	INDIA	5	4	0.0	0	09/05/1987	9
SEARO	INDONESIA	0	1	0.0	0	21/04/1987	1
SEARO	KOREA, DPR	0	0	0.0	0	10/05/1988	0*
SEARO	MALDIVES	0	0	0.0	0	30/06/1987	0
SEARO	MONGOLIA	0	0	0.0	0	31/12/1987	0
SEARO	NEPAL	0	0	0.0	0	09/05/1987	0
SEARO	SRI LANKA	1	1	0.0	0	27/05/1987	2
SEARO	THAILAND	6	6	0.0	0	12/10/1987	12
	Total for the Region	12	12	0.0	0		24

Western Pacific Region

Region	Country	1979-1986 Cases	1987 Cases	1987 Rate(a)	1988 Cases to date	Last Report	Cumulative Cases
WPRO	AUSTRALIA	387	340	2.1	86	11/04/1988	813
WPRO	BRUNEI DARUSSALAM	0	0	0.0	0	31/01/1988	0
WPRO	CHINA	1	1	0.0	0	08/09/1987	2
WPRO	CHINA (TAIWAN)	0	0	0.0	0	26/01/1988	1
WPRO	COOK ISLANDS	0	0	0.0	0	08/09/1987	0
WPRO	FIJI	0	1	0.1	0	08/09/1987	1
WPRO	FRENCH POLYNESIA	1	0	0.0	1	08/09/1987	2
WPRO	HONG KONG	3	6	0.1	3	26/01/1988	12*
WPRO	JAPAN	25	34	0.0	7	19/01/1988	66
WPRO	KIRIBATI	0	0	0.0	0	18/01/1988	0
WPRO	KOREA, REP.	0	1	0.0	1	03/03/1988	2*
WPRO	MALAYSIA	1	1	0.0	1	31/01/1988	3
WPRO	MARIANA ISLANDS	0	0	0.0	0	05/08/1987	0
WPRO	NEW CALEDONIA	0	0	0.0	1	05/08/1987	1
WPRO	NEW ZEALAND	33	30	0.9	14	30/04/1988	77*
WPRO	PAPUA NEW GUINEA	3	9	0.3	1	08/09/1987	13*
WPRO	PHILIPPINES	0	1	0.0	0	07/04/1988	1
WPRO	SAMOA	0	0	0.0	0	08/09/1987	0
WPRO	SINGAPORE	2	2	0.1	0	08/09/1987	4*
WPRO	SOLOMON ISLANDS	0	0	0.0	0	08/09/1987	0
WPRO	TONGA	0	0	0.0	1	06/10/1987	0
WPRO	TUVALU	0	0	0.0	0	08/09/1987	0*
WPRO	VANUATU	0	0	0.0	0	31/03/1988	0*
WPRO	VIET NAM	0	0	0.0	0	08/09/1987	0
	Total for the Region	456	426		113		995

** An inversion was made between Korea, DPR and Korea, REP. in the last report.
The present figures are correct.

Source: "Update: Acquired Immunodeficiency Syndrome,
31 May 1988," World Health Organization

experts. Because AIDS strikes the most productive members of society (those aged 20 to 49), and due to the drastic health problems it causes and its fatal consequences, many observers fear that those areas most heavily infected will suffer significant declines in national income. The effect on families is potentially devastating. More and more children stand to lose one or more parent, if they themselves survive. The World Health Organization's Child Survival Program, active in areas such as these which already have high infant and child mortality rates, is already considering the impact of AIDS on their program. Other development agencies have also started addressing the impact AIDS will have on such programs as immunization, breast feeding (a known source of transmission), and population programs.

Uganda - A Land Besieged

Uganda has been a land besieged by political turmoil for almost a generation. Tens of thousands of its citizens had been either killed or exiled by its ruthless dictator, Idi Amin, until his fall. Amin's fall has been followed by civil war. Struggling to rebuild after decades of slaughter and mass relocation, Uganda is once again under siege by the deadly epidemic of AIDS. Uganda is in the heart of equatorial Africa, fairly densely populated, particularly those townships along the trans-Africa highway leading to the Indian Ocean. Studies of long-distance truck drivers who travel this route have found that 33 percent of them are infected with the virus, and, likely, are contributing to the spread of the disease. Civil disturbances which lead to the displacement of large populations are also important transmission factors.

The first cases of AIDS were suspected in late 1982. Several businessmen died in an isolated fishing village known for its smuggling and illicit trading. Fellow traders called the deaths "witchcraft." Still others felt they received their just desert for being unfaithful to their wives. All were young, sexually-active, and were gone from home a great deal. The wives of these men also died mysteriously.

Soon it became clear that a new disease had hit. The caseload skyrocketed from 17 in 1983 to over 1,000 by 1987, mainly still confined to young, sexually active people. Eight out of ten cases were among people aged 20 through 40 and virtually no cases occurred among those between the ages of 5 and 14 or among the elderly. Latest statistics show an increase among those under age 5, an indication of mother-to-child transmission.

Coping

In World Health, (Geneva: World Health Organization March 1988, p. 21) Dr. Samuel I. Okware, Director of the AIDS Control Programme, Ministry of Health of Uganda, reports that AIDS in Uganda is basically an urban disease, and rarely found in rural villages where strict moral codes forbid casual sexual relationships. A study of mothers at a prenatal clinic found that 13 percent were infected with the virus, usually as a result of sexual transmission.

This epidemic is considered a social and medical disaster in a country where tuberculosis and other diseases, and the infant mortality rates were already increasing. The consequence of large numbers of AIDS deaths among the productive population threaten agricultural production and development efforts.

A National Committee for the Prevention of AIDS (NCPA) has been formed, but at present has only an advisory role in helping to formulate policy. Television and radio messages urge listeners to "love carefully" and to participate in "zero grazing," an implication that people, like cattle, should stay in their own pastures. For those communities with little access to media, political and church groups pass on the messages about AIDS. To soften the hard reality of AIDS, educators sometimes must campaign with light jokes and comic plays by theater groups.

Special efforts have been made in the areas of blood transfusion. Initial high rates of infection in donated blood meant that between 5 and 15 percent of those who had received transfusions were likely to be infected. At first, only the capital, Kampala, had limited screening facilities, but by May 1987, 13 centers had been set up around the country.

Culture and customs, far different from those of the Western world, effect research and prevention methods. Research projects include surveying social and behavioral customs, virological research, and clinical trials of local herbal remedies. Caution is used when advocating condom use until local cultural practices and attitudes are better understood. Dr. Okware reports that while little can be done for the patients, attempts are being made to improve their care and lessen their pain. They rely on psychological and spiritual counseling with the help of the church.

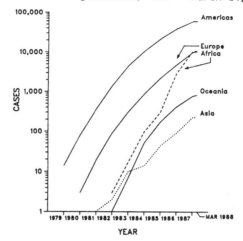

Total AIDS cases reported to the World Health Organization, 1979 – March 21, 1988

. **AIDS cases reported to the World Health Organization (WHO), by continent, 1979 – March 21, 1988**

Continent	Number of Cases	Number of Countries or Territories Reporting		Total Number of Countries Reporting
		No Cases	1 or More Cases	
Africa	10,973	8	42	50
Americas	61,602	2	42	44
Asia	231	16	21	37
Europe	10,616	1	27	28
Oceania	834	10	4	14
Total	84,256	37	136	173

AIDS cases, by age group and sex — 28 countries in the World Health Organization's European Region, December 31, 1987

Age Group	Male	Female	Total	(%)
0–11 mos	40	48	88	(0.9)
1–4 yrs	52	48	100	(1.0)
5–9 yrs	24	7	31	(0.3)
10–14 yrs	29	3	32	(0.3)
15–19 yrs	77	14	91	(0.9)
20–29 yrs	2,325	551	2,876	(28.2)
30–39 yrs	3,440	255	3,695	(36.3)
40–49 yrs	2,031	72	2,103	(20.7)
50–59 yrs	736	53	789	(7.7)
≥ 60 yrs	281	52	333	(3.3)
Unknown	38	2	43*	(0.4)
Total	9,073	1,105	10,181	(100.0)

*Sex of three patients is unknown.

Reported AIDS cases among adult and pediatric patients, by transmission category — Europe, December 31, 1987, and United States, January 4, 1988*

Transmission Categories of Patients	Europe		United States	
	No.	(%)	No.	(%)
Adult Patients				
Homosexual/Bisexual Male	5,865	(59)	32,138	(65)
Intravenous (IV) Drug Use	1,944	(20)	8,511	(17)
Homosexual Male and IV Drug Use	259	(3)	3,726	(8)
Hemophilia/Coagulation Disorder	349	(4)	494	(1)
Heterosexual Contact	609	(6)	1,987	(4)
Transfusion	359	(4)	1,144	(2)
Other/Undetermined	545	(5)	1,515	(3)
Total	9,930	(100)	49,515	(100)
Pediatric Patients				
Hemophilia/Coagulation Disorder	38	(15)	40	(5)
Parent with/at Risk for AIDS	170	(68)	577	(77)
Transfusion	38	(15)	99	(13)
Other/Undetermined	5	(2)	34	(5)
Total	251	(100)	750	(100)

*The latest data analysis available for Europe is for December 31, 1987. The January 4, 1988, U.S. analysis is used here because it most closely approximates the time frame of the European analysis.

Source: <u>Morbidity and Mortality Weekly Report</u>, May 13, 1988

EUROPE

The French Method

Professor Alain Pompidou, AIDS Counselor for the Ministry of Health, France, in World Health (March 1988), the official publication of the World Health Organization, has outlined France's five-point policy to counter the spread of AIDS which include: prevention (including information, legal measures and screening); training; monitoring and treatment; research; and international cooperation.

Prevention

In April 1987, the French government began a four-part national AIDS campaign. This program included a series of television commercials declaring that AIDS could be avoided and that it was everyone's job to stop the spread; a data base designed by the French Committee for the Education of Health, which makes daily information available to physicians through a computerized telephone system; one million copies of a booklet targeted for health professionals, and 13 million copies of a brochure for the general public; and a billboard campaign complemented by radio commercials.

Intervention among high risk groups (prisoners, drug addicts, and teenagers) will come only after special teams have been formed among those who normally come into contact with these groups. Medical staff in hospitals receive in-depth training in order to work with HIV-infected patients.

The French government has not yet adopted legal measures regarding AIDS, but some legal measures have been taken to limit the spread of the disease. These include legislation permitting the advertising of condoms (or sheaths as they are called in France), and the sale of syringes. As a one year experiment, people can buy syringes at a drugstore without either a prescription or an identification check. While the government has not halted its fight against drug abuse, it also has a fight on its hands against AIDS. An estimated 60 to 80 percent of France's heroin addicts are HIV-infected.

France has not introduced a mandatory, systematic screening, primarily due to the high cost. Instead, voluntary screening is available with respect of privacy and medical confidence. The epidemiological centers receive only coded data. Approximately 200 centers are available nationwide for screening and testing confirmation. Social Security reimburses 65 percent of the cost. Eventually free and anonymous testing will be carried out in 100 other centers. Screening is encouraged for those in high risk groups and for all couples likely to have children. Screening is mandatory for all blood, organ, tissue, cell and sperm donors. Following the recommendation of WHO and the Council of European Health Ministers, no screening of international travelers is undertaken at the border.

The Soviet Method

As of August 1987, the Soviet Union has adopted measures against AIDS which includes mandatory testing of anyone officials suspect of carrying the AIDS virus, a prison term of up to five years for exposing someone else to the virus, and a sentence of up to eight years for knowingly transmitting the virus. Anyone resisting testing could be brought in by the police. The law is aimed primarily at prostitutes and preventing them from returning to work after testing positive.

Although Soviet officials have treated the disease as almost totally a Western problem (and have maintained that it was only a minor problem in the Soviet Union), they have been speaking more openly about the disease in the past year and several diagnostic centers have opened up around the country. Television messages have been aired aimed at young people urging condom use as a preventative method, quite a departure from "normal" Soviet standards. Messages also refer vaguely to "chaste behavior."

In September 1987, general testing of foreigners began. The British Embassy reported that 41 British students were tested upon their arrival. Several African students who had tested positive were sent home. While resident businessmen and diplomats have not been tested yet, many feel it is just a matter of time.

SOUTH AMERICA

With the announcement that he and his two brothers, all hemophiliacs, were carriers of the AIDS virus, noted sociologist, Herbert de Souza broke the silence that has surrounded Brazil's more than 2,000 AIDS patients. His two brothers were well-known artists. Virtually all other AIDS victims have sought anonymity. Mr. de Souza publicly confronted the Brazilian government over their refusal to approve the importation of the antiviral drug azidothymidine (AZT), that has been shown to prolong the lives on some AIDS patients. He sought the drug for a dying friend and one of his brothers.

The Brazilian government has been harshly criticized for failure to insure a safe blood supply. Although testing began in 1985, by that time over half of Brazil's 6,000 hemophiliacs were infected - a situation not unlike that in the U.S. However, it is believed that as many as 70 percent of that country's blood banks are currently ignoring the government mandate to screen blood. The urgency of the problem can be seen in the fact that, while 2 or 3 percent of total AIDS cases in the U.S., Britain, and France are the result of blood transfusions, they account for 14 percent in Brazil. In Rio de Janeiro, they account for close to 18 percent. Some senior health officials add to the controversy by considering AIDS far less a health problem than several other diseases such as malaria and leprosy.

ASIA

As mentioned earlier, the AIDS virus has only recently arrived in Asia. Doctors at the First International Congress on AIDS in Asia in Manila in November 1987, warned that a popular notion that Asians may somehow be genetically immune to the virus was unfounded. One spokesman attributed the low incidence to luck and geography. Many Asian experts believe that transmission will more than likely reflect that of Africa and be through the heterosexual population. One spokesman reported that Asia is where the U.S. was 10 to 15 years ago.

Physicians report the entry of AIDS into the Philippines was, in many cases, the result of prostitutes having had sex with U.S. servicemen near two large American bases. By November 1987, 44 prostitutes in areas near the bases had tested positive for the AIDS virus, though none had yet shown symptoms of the disease.

In an effort to stop AIDS before it gets into the country, the People's Republic of (Mainland) China has imposed strict measures, including blood tests for foreigners and Chinese who return from abroad. Police have also stepped up efforts to prevent casual sexual encounters between Chinese and foreigners.

The forced testing by the Chinese government has been resisted by many visiting Americans, especially teachers and students who view testing as an invasion of their privacy. One American couple, teachers in their 60's, refused the test, but were allowed to stay. Western doctors have warned that taking the test may put one at danger. Many say that sterilization methods in China are haphazard, at best, and that there is risk of contracting hepatitis from infected needles. One Canadian claims to have become infected with AIDS as a result of unclean needles during acupuncture. The Chinese deny the charges.

PREVENTION AND EDUCATION

The World Health Organization believes that the spread of AIDS can only be contained through the coordinated efforts of all countries. Relying on voluntary contributions of member governments above and beyond their regular WHO contributions, WHO spent $25 million in 1987 and plans to spend $68.4 million in 1988.

The U.S. Agency for International Development (AID), is working through WHO to develop a strong program. In FY86, AID allocated $2 million to the WHO program. In FY87, the agency spent $14 million for worldwide AIDS control, including $5 million to the WHO program, $3 million to finance expected additional requests for condoms, and $6 million for technical support of bilateral prevention and control programs. The Continuing Appropriations Act of 1988 (PL 100-202) appropriated $30 million for activities related to international AIDS control, of which $14 million would go to the World Health Organization and the Pan American Health Program.

CHAPTER X

COSTS, CARE, AND CURES

In Confronting AIDS (National Academy Press, WDC, 1987), the National Academy of Sciences' Institute of Medicine wrote that the direct costs of AIDS were twofold: the personal medical care expenditures and the nonpersonal expenditures. Personal medical care expenditures include hospital services; physician care, both for inpatient and outpatient services; nursing home; home care; and hospice services. (Naturally, not all AIDS patients make use of all these facilities.) Nonpersonal expenditures include biomedical research, education campaigns, screening and testing of blood, and other support services. While the quality of care increases, although in some areas it has become incredibly overburdened, there is no cure.

WHAT DOES IT REALLY COST?

Confronting AIDS: Update 1988 (National Academy Press, WDC, 1988) estimates the average lifetime medical costs for each AIDS case to be between $55,000 and $77,000 in 1986 dollars, (from $65,000 to $80,000 in 1987 dollars) figuring from the time of diagnosis to the time of death. These are considerably lower than some earlier estimates of $147,000 for lifetime hospital costs. The difference could be that experience has shown that there are alternatives to lifetime hospital confinement. One team of experts, including A. A. Scitovsky and D. P. Rice ("Estimates of the direct and indirect costs of acquired immunodeficiency in the United States, 1985, 1986, and 1991." Public Health Reports 102:5-17) estimates that in current dollars, the total direct costs for AIDS in 1986 was $1.64 billion. The bulk of the costs, $1.1 billion, went for personal care, while the remaining $542 million was spent for nonpersonal costs. At this point, however, cost estimates appear to be just that, estimates. Prices can vary widely on everything from methods of treatment to where the AIDS patient gets that treatment.

Due to fewer and shorter hospital stays, hospital treatment costs for AIDS patients have declined. Different methods of handling AIDS patients have undoubtedly brought this about. During the beginning years of the AIDS epidemic, patients were more likely to be placed in intensive care units than they are now. San Francisco, because of its early attention to AIDS and AIDS patients, has probably done the best of any area in developing and mobilizing outpatient and community support groups which alleviate a lot of the need for long hospital stays and thereby drastically reducing medical costs. Presently, these and similar outreach programs throughout the country depend on unpaid labor. If the epidemic spreads as public health officials predict, the volunteer pool will probably shrink. In many instances, the volunteers are themselves potential patients. If volunteers are replaced by professional help, home care could become as expensive as institutional care.

Future Costs

Based on the CDC projection of 172,800 AIDS patients by 1991, Scitovsky and Rice estimate the total annual costs to be $66.5 billion. Of these, $8.5 billion would be for personal expenditures, $2.3 billion for nonpersonal expenses, and $55.6 billion for indirect costs. Indirect costs include loss of wages due to illness and disability and the loss of future wages because of premature death. The loss in future productivity is expected to be substantial, because the disease primarily strikes young adults who are in their most productive years. In 1986, the direct cost of AIDS represented 0.4 percent of the total U.S. health expenditures; by 1991, it is expected to reach approximately 1.5 percent of total national health expenditures.

While that proportion will still be relatively small in 1991, it will not be evenly distributed across the country. Certain metropolitan areas, already economically overburdened, will be hit the hardest. At the end of 1986, San Francisco and New York City housed 34 percent of this country's AIDS cases. During that same year AIDS patients occupied approximately 3 percent of all medical/surgical beds in each of these two cities, while nationally, AIDS patients only occupied 0.4 percent of all beds. By 1991, the figures are expected to rise to 8.1 percent for New York, 12.4 percent for San Francisco, and 1.9 percent nationally. In 1986, AIDS inpatient treatment costs for New York were 3.1 percent of the total inpatient costs; in San Francisco, 3.5 percent; and nationally 0.6 percent. By 1991, the costs could rise to 8.4 percent, 16.2 percent, and 3 percent, respectively.

Who Pays?

The Health Care Financing Administration of the U.S. Department Of Health and Human Services (HHS) estimates that 40 percent of all AIDS patients are served under Medicaid (a health program for persons who qualify whose income is below the poverty level). In locations most greatly effected, such as New York and New Jersey, as many as 65 to 70 percent of AIDS patients may be on Medicaid. Federal and state expenditures for AIDS patients in 1988 is expected to reach $600 million, and rise to $1.8 billion by 1991. D.P. Andrulis, et.al., in "The provision and financing of medical care for AIDS patients in U.S. public and private teaching hospitals" (Journal of the American Medical Association, Vol. 258:1343-1346, 1987), reported that a survey of 169 public and private teaching hospitals found 54 percent of AIDS cases were covered by Medicaid, while 17 percent were covered by private insurance. When public hospitals were considered separately, 62 percent were Medicaid-covered, while only 7 percent had private insurance.

AIDS and Health Insurers

The Office of Technology Assessment, the fact-finding arm of the U.S. Congress, surveyed the response of health insurers to the AIDS epidemic in AIDS and Health Insurance: A Survey (WDC, 1988). Commercial carriers cover 9.3 million people; Blue Cross and Blue Shield (BC/BS) plans cover 4.2 million; and Health Maintenance Organizations cover 1 million. Approximately 14.5 million non-Medicare individuals and their families have health insurance that is not part of one of the above group memberships. It is these individuals and their carriers who were the focus of this survey. They must meet certain underwriting standards to be covered by health insurance. Applicants and their attending physicians must answer pertinent questions regarding their medical history, and health insurers consider a question concerning the presence of AIDS antibody a logical and essential part of this overall risk assessment.

--Commercial Insurers, BC/BS Plans, and HMOs Attempting to Identify
Individual Applicants Exposed to the AIDS Virus

Attempt to identify applicants exposed to the AIDS virus	Commercial insurers[a] (n=59)		BC/BS plans (n=15)		HMOs (n=15)	
	Number	Percent	Number	Percent	Number	Percent
Yes.............................	41	69.5% ┐	8	53% ┐	8	53%
		86%		73%		
No, but plans to.................	10	16.9 ┘	3	20 ┘	0	--
No, and no plans to[b]...........	8	14	2	13	6	40
Other, including:						
-AIDS policies under review....	0	--	1	7	1	7
-Yes, but for less than .5% of applicants......	0	--	1	7	0	--

[a]Two insurers did not answer this question.
[b]Three HMOs are prohibited by State law from medical screening of any kind.

SOURCE: Office of Technology Assessment, 1988.

--Commercial Insurers, BC/BS Plans, and HMOs
Methods Used to Screen Individual Applicants for Exposure to the AIDS Virus

Method(s) used to identify AIDS exposure	Commercial insurers[a] (n=51)		BC/BS plans[a] (n=11)		HMOs[a] (n=8)	
	Number	Percent	Number	Percent	Number	Percent
Question on application..........	44	86%	11	100%	8	100%
Attending physician statement.....	42	82	9	82	6	75
ELISA and western blot...........	31	61	1	9	2	25
T-Cell subset study..............	17	33	0	--	0	0
Other, including: physical exam if high risk....	0	--	0	--	1	13

[a]Data include only those insurers or plans that screen or intend to screen for AIDS exposure.

SOURCE: Office of Technology Assessment, 1988.

Of those who responded to the survey, 86 percent of the commercial insurers, 73 percent of the BC/BS plans, and 53 percent of the HMOs, either
attempt to identify applicants exposed to the AIDS virus or have intentions to
start asking this question soon. The most common method of screening is by
incorporating a question on the health history portion of the application.
Only seven companies that asked screening questions did not use an AIDS question. Generally, the companies have included this question so they can use it
later to contest a pre-existing condition. For example, if an applicant
knowingly does not tell the truth about HIV positive, AIDS symptoms or fully
diagnosed AIDS or ARC, the insurer has grounds for denying reimbursement.
Sixty-one percent of commercial companies, 9 percent of BC/BS plans, and 25
percent of HMOs use ELISA and Western blot tests for screening.

Tightening Restrictions

In addition to the steps already taken, many companies plan other measures. The most common plans involve introducing tighter underwriting guidelines so that the market shrinks, and expanding HIV and other testing. Other
plans include placing a dollar limit on AIDS coverage and establishing a
waiting period for AIDS benefits.

--Response to the AIDS Epidemic:
Reported Plans by Commercial Health Insurers, BC/BS Plans, and HMOs

Reported Plans	Commercial insurers (n=61)		BC/BS plans (n=15)		HMOs (n=16)	
	Number	Percent	Number	Percent	Number	Percent
Withdraw from the individual health market altogether[a]	0	--	0	--	1	6%
Exclude AIDS and/or sexually transmitted diseases from individual health coverage	5	8%	1	7%	0	--
Reduce company exposure in the individual and small group health markets (e.g., by introducing more restrictive underwriting guidelines)	21	34	6	40	5	31
Expand HIV or other testing of applicants	20	33	1	7	2	13
Terminate open enrollment	NA[b]	--	0	--	0	--
Other:						
- Considering one or more of the above	3	5	0	--	0	--
- Would consider any of the above policies if they were adopted by competing HMOs	NA	--	NA	--	1	6
- Add an AIDS question to application	9	15	2	13	0	--
- Include a dollar limit for AIDS care in new policies	2	3	0	--	0	--
- Establish a 12-24 waiting month period for AIDS	1	2	0	--	0	--
- Deny applicants with a history of sexually transmitted disease and expand waiting period for hepatitis, lymph disease, and mononucleosis	0	--	1	7	0	--
- Expand education role	0	--	2	7	0	--
- Policies currently under review	0	--	2	13	2	13
- Considering HIV testing	0	--	0	--	1	6
No actions planned or reported	10	16	2	13	7	44

[a]One commercial insurer reported withdrawing from the Washington, D.C. market.
[b]NA=Not Applicable.

SOURCE: Office of Technology Assessment, 1988.

Of the 61 commercial insurers who responded to the survey, 45, had reimbursed at least one individual policyholder for AIDS-related care. A total of 1,010 AIDS cases were reported, and the average insurer cared for 22 AIDS-related cases. Bear in mind that surveillance of AIDS-related cases is sketchy at best. BC/BS, also acknowledging sketchy surveillance, had nationwide caseloads which varied in AIDS-related cases ranging from 1 to 3,000 subscribers who were reimbursed for AIDS-related care. Geography played a large part in the disparity. Those BC/BS caseloads in the Northeast were more likely to have subscribers with AIDS.

Some States Prohibit Tightening of Restrictions

In 1986, the District of Columbia passed a sweeping insurance anti-discrimination law preventing the sale of any life or health insurance plan that required HIV antibody testing or proof of testing. The new law applied to test restrictions for five years at which point the insurers could apply to increase rates based upon the results of a test used to screen or test for AIDS. The test required the approval of the commission of Public Health. The law does not apply to new applicants who have been diagnosed as having AIDS by a physician. In October 1986, a federal judge upheld the law, and an estimated 32 insurance companies stopped writing individual health and life insurance policies in D.C.

In August 1987, the New York State Superintendent of Insurance issued a regulation barring insurers from requiring health insurance applicants to take the test for the the virus that causes AIDS. Not unexpectedly, the state's insurers, with the exception of Empire Blue Cross and Blue Shield which does not require testing, vehemently opposed the prohibition, citing their fear for their solvency and their concern for the majority of their policyholders who were not engaged in high risk behavior. The insurers are not required to cover those with AIDS, or ARC. California recently enacted a similar law.

Number of AIDS-related cases	Number of companies (n=51)a	Percent of companies reporting AIDS-related experience
None	6	12%
1-10	28	55
11-49	13	25
50-100	2	4
More than 100 ...	2	4

a Ten of the sixty-one respondents (16%) were unable to provide AIDS-related case data.

SOURCE: Office of Technology Assessment, 1988.

FEDERAL SPENDING ON AIDS

Many feel that the Reagan Administration was unnecessarily slow in releasing funds for AIDS research and treatment. When AIDS became known in 1981, no new funding was made available by the Administration or the Congress. During the same time period, Toxic Shock Syndrome, a mostly fatal condition linked to tampon use, and the Legionnaire's Disease, a peculiar fatal condition

--Blue Cross/Blue Shield Plans
Number of Subscribers Reimbursed for AIDS-Related Claims

	No open enrollment (n=10)	Open enrollment (n=5)a	All plans (n=15)
Total number of subscribers reimbursed for AIDS-related claimsb......................	453	3,480	3,933 c
Number of plans reporting AIDS-related claims..........	7 (70%)	3 (60%)	10 (67%)
Average number of AIDS-related cases per plan........	65	1,160	393

aOne of the five plans holds a limited open enrollment period; the others are continuous.
bAIDS-related claims data reflect both individual and group policy experience.
cOne plan alone reported 3,000 subscribers with AIDS; the other plans had an average AIDS-related caseload of 104.

SOURCE: Office of Technology Assessment, 1988.

which affected members of the American Legion at a Philadelphia Hotel, sparked much public interest and many public dollars. Critics of Administration policy believe that because those involved in the early years of AIDS were homosexual males, and later drug users, the public was not as concerned, and the media was reluctant to report, so the Administration and the Congress felt no need to act.

An Increase, But Still Not Enough

Federal funding for AIDS has grown from a pittance of $200,000 in FY81 (all funds redirected from other projects) to over $951 million in FY88, a sum many AIDS researchers still find inadequate. Until Congress appropriated money for AIDS research in FY83, all funds were redirected from other Health and Human Services (HHS) agencies. The Centers for Disease Control (CDC), which did much of the basic "grunt" work in the early days (and still works diligently in AIDS research and surveillance) was severely understaffed and underfunded. On the other hand, the National Institute of Cancer (NIC), where Dr. Robert Gallo discovered HTLV-III, the virus which causes AIDS, has always been well funded.

Since the first Congressional funding in FY83, the budget for AIDS research and education has been increasing by large percentages every year. The

FUNCTIONAL BREAKDOWN OF PHS SPENDING ON AIDS
(in thousands of dollars)

	FY84 Actual	FY85 Actual	FY86 Actual	FY87 Actual	FY88 Approp. a/	FY89 Request
I. Pathogenesis and Clinical Manifestations	$45,690	$61,051	$90,257	$154,423	$276,279	$385,571
II. Therapeutics	8,728	11,950	58,180	129,061	175,727	243,244
III. Vaccines	2,879	10,186	18,049	33,210	62,259	92,611
IV. Public Health Control Measures (total)	4,081	25,222	51,712	145,040	315,351	400,097
A. Information/Education	1,423	6,541	28,440	132,539	296,355	373,567
1. General Public (non-add)	(749)	(3,238)	(5,206)	(28,519)	(49,546)	(50,785)
2. School & College Age (non-add)	---	(136)	(114)	(11,076)	(29,916)	(36,450)
3. High Risk & Infected Persons (non-add)	(282)	(2,549)	(20,211)	(81,970)	(189,525)	(241,970)
a. Testing/counseling/referral (non-add)	---	---	(218)	(26,039)	(72,493)	(102,738)
4. Health Care Workers (non-add)	(392)	(618)	(2,909)	(10,974)	(27,368)	(44,362)
B. Prevention of Transfusion-related AIDS	522	11,531	11,650	1,733	3,040	3,312
C. Development & Evaluation of Blood Tests	2,136	7,150	11,622	10,768	15,956	23,218
V. Patient Care and Health Care Needs	82	209	15,595	40,721	29,218	67,731
VI. Multidisciplinary Research	---	---	---	---	92,205	95,746
A. Construction					(43,085)	(25,000)
VII. Contingency Funds	---	---	---	---	---	15,000
TOTAL, PUBLIC HEALTH SERVICE	$61,460	$108,618	$233,793	$502,455	$951,039	$1,300,000

a/ This total includes two amounts not shown in the AIDS tables of the FY88 conference agreement (H.Rept. 100-498): $19,150 of the construction money (in the NIH B&F account), and $660 additional for NIH (in the NIAMS account).

Source: Public Health Service Budget Office, Mar. 25, 1988.

FY88 apportionment of $951,039,000 was 89 percent more than the FY87 figure of $502,455,000. The proposed FY89 budget allocated $1.3 billion, a 37 percent increased over the previous year. Many observers and critics believe that had funding been more realistic in the early years, many deaths could have been prevented and researchers would be that much closer to a cure or a vaccine.

FY83 and FY84, A Beginning

In 1982, CDC spent, $2 million; the FDA, $150,000; and the National Institutes of Health, $3.4 million, for a total outlay of $5.6 million by the Public Health Service. No special appropriation for AIDS research, treatment, or education had been made. By the time appropriations came in FY83, over 1,000 persons had died from AIDS.

Following considerable floor debate, President Reagan signed into law a FY83 supplemental appropriations bill (PL 98-63) providing an extra $12.6 million for AIDS research. The NIH received the bulk of the monies ($9 million), while the CDC received $2.23 million.

The revised FY84 budget provided $39.8 million for funding research for AIDS, up from the original Reagan budget request of only $17.6 million. The additional $22.2 million was to be transferred from other agencies, such as the National Health Services Corps field program and the Rural Development Loan program. Of the additional monies, CDC would get $7.3 million and NIH, $14.9 million. It was still a robbing Peter to pay Paul set up. In October 1983,

FUNCTIONAL BREAKDOWN OF PHS SPENDING ON AIDS
(in thousands of dollars)

	FY84 Actual	FY85 Actual	FY86 Actual	FY87 Actual	FY88 Approp. a/	FY89 Request
I. Pathogenesis and Clinical Manifestations	$45,690	$61,051	$90,257	$154,423	$276,279	$385,571
II. Therapeutics	8,728	11,950	58,180	129,061	175,727	243,244
III. Vaccines	2,879	10,186	18,049	33,210	62,259	92,611
IV. Public Health Control Measures (total)	4,081	25,222	51,712	145,040	315,351	400,097
A. Information/Education	1,423	6,541	28,440	132,539	296,355	373,567
1. General Public (non-add)	(749)	(3,238)	(5,206)	(28,519)	(49,546)	(50,785)
2. School & College Age (non-add)	---	(136)	(114)	(11,076)	(29,916)	(36,450)
3. High Risk & Infected Persons (non-add)	(282)	(2,549)	(20,211)	(81,970)	(189,525)	(241,970)
a. Testing/counseling/referral (non-add)	---	---	(218)	(26,039)	(72,493)	(102,738)
4. Health Care Workers (non-add)	(392)	(618)	(2,909)	(10,974)	(27,368)	(44,362)
B. Prevention of Transfusion-related AIDS	522	11,531	11,650	1,733	3,040	3,312
C. Development & Evaluation of Blood Tests	2,136	7,150	11,622	10,768	15,956	23,218
V. Patient Care and Health Care Needs	82	209	15,595	40,721	29,218	67,731
VI. Multidisciplinary Research	---	---	---	---	92,205	95,746
A. Construction					(43,085)	(25,000)
VII. Contingency Funds	---	---	---	---	---	15,000
TOTAL, PUBLIC HEALTH SERVICE	$61,460	$108,618	$233,793	$502,455	$951,039	$1,300,000

a/ This total includes two amounts not shown in the AIDS tables of the FY88 conference agreement (H.Rept. 100-498): $19,150 of the construction money (in the NIH B&F account), and $660 additional for NIH (in the NIAMS account).

Source: Public Health Service Budget Office, Mar. 25, 1988.

NIH EXPENDITURES FOR AIDS RESEARCH
(in thousands of dollars)

Institute	FY82 Actual	FY83 Actual	FY84 Actual	FY85 Actual	FY86 Actual	FY87 Actual	FY88 Approp.	FY89 Request
Cancer	$2,400	$9,790	$16,627	$26,874	$45,050	$63,755	$89,944	$125,280
Heart, Lung, & Blood	5	1,202	4,871	9,323	15,468	17,244	24,738	39,032
Dental	25	25	81	97	1,712	3,247	3,169	3,526
Diabetes, Digestive, & Kidney Diseases	---	---	---	---	---	495	3,351	3,650
Neurological	31	684	1,510	1,168	1,435	3,685	12,212	13,393
Allergy & Infectious Diseases	297	9,223	19,616	23,273	63,276	145,760	223,383	310,268
Gen'l Med. Sciences	---	---	---	---	---	5,420	2,394	11,100
Child Health & Human Development	---	---	---	---	1,400	4,762	14,292	20,443
Eye	33	45	60	200	96	253	3,830	4,947
Environmental Health Sciences	---	---	---	---	---	216	3,917	4,234
Aging	---	---	---	---	---	184	361	452
Arthritis & Musculo-skeletal & Skin	---	---	---	---	---	100	660	687
Research Resources	564	699	1,356	2,802	6,157	11,027	50,418	38,010
Nursing	---	---	---	---	---	---	510	707
Fogarty Int'l Center	---	---	---	---	---	---	4,500	4,736
Office of Director	---	---	---	---	73	4,759	10,977	7,165
Bldgs & Facilities *	---	---	---	---	---	---	19,150	---
TOTAL, NIH	$3,355	$21,668	$44,121	$63,737	$134,667	$260,907	$467,806	$587,630

* The B&F funds were not included in the AIDS tables of the FY88 conference agreement on the continuing resolution, but report language indicates that the funds will be used for facility renovation related to AIDS on the NIH campus. AIDS funding for the Arthritis Institute also was not included in the conference agreement.

Source: PHS Budget Office and conference report on the FY88 continuing resolution, March 1988.

Congress passed PL 98-130 which allotted additional funds for AIDS research, but not for the Public Health Emergency Fund, which meant no money was being spent for education.

The Administration proposed a total Public Health Service (PHS) budget of $54.1 million for AIDS research to be divided among CDC, FDA, and the Alcohol, Drug Abuse, and Mental Health Administration. Because of the discoveries by NIC and others concerning a possible AIDS virus, the Administration wanted to revise the FY84 and FY85 figures to reflect efforts aimed at developing a blood screening method for early detection, and a vaccine. In November 1984, PL 98-619 was signed into law, authorizing $84.1 million to various PHS agencies. On July 19, 1985, after much controversy, HHS Secretary Margaret M. Heckler sent a memo to the House Appropriations Committee indicating that HHS intended to re-direct FY85 funds in order to spend additional money on AIDS. As a result, actual AIDS funding to PHS was $108.6 million, much of it redirected funds.

FY86, A Proposed Cut

President Reagan's original request for $85.6 million was a sum most observers thought not equal to fight a disease the President had dubbed "Public Enemy #1." The figure represented a decrease from the CDC and Federal Drug Administration (FDA) budget from previous year, which the President said was due to one-time costs of facility renovations and blood supply studies. In July 1985, HHS Secretary Heckler notified the House Appropriations that HHS had not only requested an additional $37.8 million, but a redirection of FY86 HHS funds to bring the PHS total to $126.5 million, almost tripling CDC's budget and giving $3 million more to the FDA.

Gramm-Rudman-Hollings

The Gramm-Rudman-Hollings Balanced Budget and Emergency Control Act of 1985 (PL99-177) required a 4.3 percent "across the board" sequestration (seizing as security for a debt) of the FY86 AIDS research budget. This caused a reduction of almost $2.8 million to the CDC budget. When the Gramm-Rudman-Hollings budget cuts are taken into account, the PHS total for FY86 was $233 million, leaving CDC with $62 million, and NIH with $134.6 million. The Administration wanted to rescind portions of the FY86 AIDS research budget in order to prepare for the necessary Gramm-Rudman-Hollings FY87 budget cuts, but both Senate and House Appropriations Subcommittees rejected these proposals. Actual FY86 funding was $233.8 million.

FY87

In a special budget document, "Major Policy Initiatives – FY87," the Administration identified AIDS research as one of its priority items. The Administration requested $231 million for AIDS research in FY87 and a single office under the Assistant Secretary of Health to plan AIDS control efforts. This was similar to Congressional appeals for an AIDS "czar." The Administration also asked that Congress "establish a single funding authority and give HHS the authority to redirect, where appropriate, up to 1 percent of funding from lower priority HHS programs to AIDS research and control." Actual funding for AIDS research and education for FY87 was $502.5 million

FY88

Congress increased the Reagan Administration's original request of $533.9 million to over $951 million. This request included $9.5 million to the CDC for an every-household mailing project which had been cut from the FY87 budget.

GOVERNMENT-WIDE SPENDING ON AIDS
(Obligations in $ millions)

	FY82 Actual	FY83 Actual	FY84 Actual	FY85 Actual	FY86 Actual	FY87 Actual	FY88 Estimate	FY89 Estimate
Public Health Service	6	29	61	109	234	502	951	1300
Medicaid (Federal share)	*	*	*	*	130	210	375	600
Social Security	*	*	*	*	*	41	71	111
Medicare	*	*	*	*	*	10	15	25
Veterans	2	5	6	12	24	30	52	66
Defense	0	0	0	0	79	74	52	52
Prisons	*	*	*	0	1	3	6	6
State	0	0	0	0	0	1	2	2
Labor	0	0	0	0	0	1	1	1
TOTAL	8	34	67	121	467	872	1525	2162

*   No estimate is available for this year.

Public Health Service -- PHS supports research into the causes, prevention, and potential cures of AIDS. Through education, PHS also attempts to prevent the further spread of AIDS.

Medicaid and Social Security Disability Insurance -- HHS deems AIDS patients to be disabled, which qualifies them for Social Security Disability Insurance (SSDI) benefits and in certain circumstances, for Supplementary Security Income (SSI) benefits. In many States, SSI eligibility may guarantee them Medicaid eligibility.

Medicare -- Some AIDS patients are over 65, some have been on Social Security Disability long enough (24 months) to qualify for Medicare, and a few qualify for other reasons.

Veterans Administration -- VA provides medical care to veterans with AIDS. The estimates for 1988-92 are subject to wide variation. This is a conservative estimate which assumes that the 1987-92 increase in cases will not exceed the 1986-87 increase.

Defense -- Defense is screening current personnel and recruits for evidence of AIDS infection. As the backlog of current personnel are screened, required funding will decline.

Bureau of Prisons -- The Bureau of Prisons randomly tests asymptomatic inmates entering Federal prisons, and uniformly tests all persons being released from Federal prisons. Medical staff treat inmates with AIDS. Beginning in FY88, all prisoners with AIDS will be offered AZT.

State Department -- State conducts AIDS antibody tests as part of routine in-service physical examinations of Foreign Service Officers and physical examinations for new employees, and has recently begun testing refugees and persons seeking immigrant visas.

Department of Labor -- DOL screens current Job Corps enrollees and new applicants for evidence of AIDS infection.

Source: Office of Management and Budget, March 17, 1988.

FY89

The FY89 request for $1.3 billion for AIDS was $349 million (37 percent) more than the FY88 request.

CARING FOR PEOPLE WITH AIDS

Caring for a person with AIDS is especially difficult because of the multi-faceted nature of AIDS. It is not one disease, but several; it often requires multiple stays in the hospital; testing often borders on invasion of privacy; and the mortality rate is very high, if not, eventually, 100 percent.

Hospital Care

Some hospitals, beset with large numbers of AIDS patients, have created centralized, special units for the purpose of AIDS care. Modeled after the original unit at San Francisco General Hospital assembled by Dr. Paul Volberding, one of the pioneers in AIDS treatment, these units are somewhat like cancer wards. Patients are cared for by nurses and support staff specially trained to deal with their sociological and psychological needs. As the demand for care increases, however, only the most serious cases may be able to use these units. Some hospitals feel care by an AIDS team is an alternative, while others believe that due to the diverse needs of AIDS patients, their care should be distributed among several attending physicians. Whatever the solution, many hospitals have become overburdened with patients. In addition, some hospitals have developed a reputation for being an "AIDS hospital," a distinction few seek, and one not likely to help attract patients with other problems.

Outpatient Care

Adequate outpatient care must also include access to inpatient facilities, since frequent stays in the hospital are almost inevitable. Outpatient care ideally is multidisciplinary, and available at an AIDS clinic. Those who specialize in the many facets of AIDS treatment, dermatology, infectious disease, oncology (cancer) and pulmonary disease, are available through the clinic, as well as those who can help the AIDS victim deal with the psychosocial problems AIDS patients often face.

Community-Based Care

Community-based care is care which an AIDS patient receives at home which supplements of replaces hospital-based care. This includes giving the medicines with the proper nursing supervision and home hospice programs which give social support in the terminal stages of the sickness.

In San Francisco, a community-based group, Shanti, which was concerned with death counseling, together with the City of San Francisco, organized the Shanti Project, to provide small-group housing for AIDS patients who would otherwise not be able to stay on their own. Several patients share apartments monitored by Shanti staff members. The patients are able to help each other to supplement the assistance they receive from the volunteers. Similar programs have sprung up throughout the country.

AIDS Among the Homeless

Despite attempts by New York City to provide special housing for homeless AIDS patients, top city health officials suspect that thousands of people with

AIDS are living in the city's homeless shelters. Many have fallen through the cracks of the health system which has not properly diagnosed them, while others do not know that they are sick. Still others hide their disease from the other shelter residents out of fear of being physically and verbally abused. Dr. Stephen C. Joseph, the city's Health Commissioner, confirms that many in the city's shelters are infected with the AIDS virus.

While others in the shelter are concerned with becoming infected by the AIDS residents, Dr. Joseph insists that those with AIDS are in greater danger since their immune systems have difficulty fighting the the potentially dangerous diseases to be found in such shelters. Many hospitals are overwhelmed with AIDS patients who literally have no place to go once they are discharged from the hospital and many will undoubtedly also end up in city shelters. Advocacy groups for AIDS patients have pressed the city for additional housing for homeless AIDS victims, which Dr. Joseph claims are forthcoming.

Mental and Emotional Support

Not surprisingly, depression is a common psychiatric problem among patients who are seriously ill with AIDS. Not just the normal grief response, this depression is a combination of feelings of alienation, guilt, lack of self-esteem, and frequently, contemplation of suicide. These feeling are often related to how the person became infected with AIDS. Therapy, antidepressant medication, and necessary precautions to prevent suicide are often necessary for treatment.

Some patients with AIDS have difficulty emerging from the denial stage of their fatal illness. They hold on to false hopes which may interfere with their medical care or they refuse to change high-risk behavior which would endanger others. They have to be forced to confront their denial and accept proper treatment and change their behavior.

In addition to coping with the numerous problem posed by AIDS - dying at a young age, weakness, pain - AIDS patients are also faced with possible ostracism from friends and family; lack of a supportive network; and inadequate facilities and funds. The real or imagined burden of having passed the infection on to others can be very heavy.

TREATMENT, CURES, AND VACCINES

There is no cure for AIDS. Treatment is limited to three areas: 1) treat the opportunistic infection or cancer in the patient; 2) treat the AIDS virus itself; 3) stimulate the person's immune system.

The first approach is only palliative (eases the pain without curing), because the disease is still there. While some drugs have proved useful in reducing or eliminating Kaposi's sarcoma lesions and other cancers, the treatment still does not help the patient regain the function of his immune system. The opportunistic infections have been particularly hard to treat.

The second approach requires the use of anti-viral agents. Although new agents are being developed, only a small number are presently available. Because viruses are parasites which make use of many of the internal mechanisms of the host cell, most drugs which inhibit the virus activity also disturb the host cell function, causing toxic effects in the patient. The complicated characteristics of the AIDS virus make it particularly difficult to halt. The virus incorporates its genetic material into that of the infected cell making it almost impossible to tell one from the other. When the host cell divides, the viral genes are reproduced. Drug therapy may never be able to completely rid the patient of the virus and he or she may require lifetime treatment to control the virus. In addition, the virus is known to infect the central nervous system and many drugs cannot cross the blood-brain barrier.

The FDA approved AZT in March 1987. The drug costs $7,000 to $10,000 annually per patient. Reportedly, the high cost and limited supply are due to the difficulty in making AZT, which takes seven months to manufacture. Effective September 1987, the Public Health Service, in cooperation with Burroughs Wellcome Company, announced azidothymidine (AZT) would be made more available to AIDS patients. AZT does not cure AIDS, but many patients have fewer serious medical complications and an improved sense of well-being. Others say it simply prolongs life for a few months, but that should be up to the AIDS patient to decide. A side effect of the drug is that it reduces the blood cell count, sometimes causing anemia so severe that patients have to be taken off the drug and given transfusions.

Other drugs which are being tested for use in the treatment of AIDS (and, in some cases, ARC) are: foscarnet, (PFA, phophonoformate), HAP-23, Virazole (ribavirin) suramin, and AL721. Several drugs which affect the immune system are also being tested: alpha interferon, gamma interferon, IMREG-1, and cycosporine. Several already have been tried on AIDS patients, but with little or no success.

Perhaps the best hope for any kind of success is treating the patient in the early stages of the disease before the immune system has been destroyed. The potentially long incubation period (sometimes as long as ten years) makes determining when to begin treatment particularly difficult. In June 1986, the National Institute of Allergy and Infectious Diseases awarded $100 million over the following five years to 14 medical centers to conduct clinical trials of drugs for this type of AIDS treatment.

Work on a Vaccine

Although research is underway on a vaccine, there are many serious difficulties. The AIDS virus mutates at approximately a hundred times the rate of other viruses. As a result, the genetic structure may vary significantly and changes rapidly. Samples of the isolated virus from different patients vary by as much as 30 percent. Therefore, a vaccine developed against one strain of the virus would not necessarily be effective against other strains.

A vaccine works because it causes the immune system to produce antibodies against the organism causing the disease. Under ordinary circumstances, these antibodies circulate in the blood system for years, protecting against further onslaught from future invasions. Although high levels of antibodies to the AIDS virus are usually found in AIDS patients, they do not seem to protect against the disease. Because of the lack of a protective or "neutralizing" antibody, some scientists wonder whether protective immunity could even be induced against this virus using an AIDS vaccine.

A third problem is that this virus can be transferred by direct contact between cells, evading detection by antibodies in the blood, which may be why the disease spreads in spite of the antibody production. In order to be successful, the vaccine might first have to interfere with the first round of infections.

Serious Problems

As with any vaccine, there are many social and legal complications. The vaccine requires testing on human subjects, requiring a volunteer test group. Testing in humans would take about three years, possibly as long as eight years, because of the long latency period. The subjects would have to be monitored for that length of time to determine the safety and effectiveness of the vaccine. Those in the test group would have to continue their high risk behavior in order to determine if the vaccine works. To make matters worse, they would be HIV positive and possibly have difficulty getting employment and insurance.

If such a vaccine were found to be safe, public health officials would have to determine who should be vaccinated. Since the majority of the population is not homosexual, or addicted to drugs, or hemophiliac, vaccinating everyone would not be practical, and probably not acceptable. Prevention through changing high risk behavior is both far more acceptable and effective.

Finally, there is the question of liability. Most pharmaceutical companies no longer manufacture vaccines, because it leaves them vulnerable to lawsuits, even if the vaccine were manufactured properly. Even if the federal government takes responsibility, the problems could be worse than those associated with the swine flu epidemic vaccine in the mid 1970s. An estimated $4 billion in claims were brought against the U.S. government as a result of mass immunization for the swine flu epidemic.

CHAPTER XI

PREVENTION AND EDUCATION

In the case of AIDS, prevention and education are closely intertwined. Since at this time neither a vaccine nor a cure for AIDS is available, the only recourse is to see that everyone is properly educated on the ways to prevent becoming infected and to prevent others from becoming infected.

QUARANTINE AND CRIME

Chapter XIII discusses the issue of quarantining infected individuals and bringing criminal charges against those who knowingly endanger other lives. While it is unlikely that the U.S. Constitution will support quarantining, there are also many other questions about the advisability and the effectiveness of bringing criminal charges against an infected individual who knows that his or her condition is terminal.

UNCONTAMINATED BLOOD

Since the introduction of the ELISA and Western blot tests in 1985, over 36 million blood or plasma donations in the United have been tested for HIV infection. The unfortunate victims of contaminated blood used before the testing cannot be helped now, but hopefully, others will now be safe. Virtually all blood donated in the U.S. is now tested for HIV antibody.

New concern over the safety of the blood supply came when it was found that HIV, the virus which causes AIDS can hide in the macrophages and not cause the T-4 cells to make antibodies. It is these antibodies which are detected by the ELISA and Western blot tests. In June 1988, the Cetus Corporation of Emeryville, California announced that it had licensed two laboratories to carry a new diagnostic test which could detect the AIDS virus even if it is hiding in the cells. The new test, called polymearse chain reaction, or PCR, amplifies minute amounts of important genetic material in the cells, making them easier to identify. Now the AIDS virus can be detected in patients who do not have antibodies to the virus. This test is not only important for the blood supply, but might be particularly useful in testing infants who are exposed to the AIDS virus perinatally, since it is often difficult to determine whether the child has been infected for the first 15 months of its life.

AMONG DRUG ABUSERS

While the incidence of AIDS among homosexual men appears to be dropping, the incidence among drug abusers is growing. Intravenous drug abusers are often those who have given up on many aspects of life and the quality of whose life has dropped to little more than nothing. Though there are some drug abusers who sincerely want help through counseling and rehabilitation, others cannot or will not change. Attempts to educate these abusers about protecting the safety of others is predicated on the often erroneous assumption that they even care about their own safety.

One of the more controversial methods of prevention among drug abusers has been the issuance of clean syringes, since sharing of dirty needles is a major way of spreading the infection. While the ideal situation would be for IV drug users to abandon drug use, or at best, switch to noninjectable drugs, this is unlikely. At least four countries - The Netherlands, the United Kingdom, Australia, and Switzerland - have started experimenting with free, government supported needle exchange programs. At a 1987 World Health Organization meeting, The Netherlands reported that, as a result of their program, needle sharing had declined from 75 percent to 25 percent from 1985 to 1987.

No consensus has been reached in the U.S. about supplying clean needles for drug users. However, areas of the Northeast, which have been hit hardest by AIDS among drug abusers, have begun experimenting with such programs. Not only do they hope it will stop the spread of AIDS, but that it will help attract the addicts to treatment clinics and programs. In New York, drug users who participate in the program will receive clean needles in exchange for attending therapy sessions. The experimental New York program will begin with 200 to 400 participants, but hopefully increase to several thousand. New York has over 250,000 intravenous drug users, half of whom are infected with AIDS.

AIDS AND CONDOMS

Even more controversial than the clean needle program is the advertisement and endorsement of condoms as a means of preventing the spread of AIDS. Compared to many European nations, the U.S. has a reputation for being uncomfortable about the discussion of sex. The idea of a television or radio commercial discussing the use of condoms was unthinkable even a decade ago, and still causes raised eyebrows and some protest. However, the nation has never been faced with a situation like AIDS before, made all the more difficult because it requires discussion of sex, and more specifically, sex among homosexuals. However, AIDS is no longer considered the "gay" disease, and use of condoms to prevent heterosexual as well as homosexual transmission has become more and more accepted.

Under laboratory conditions, condoms have been proven to obstruct the transmittal of HIV virus. Natural membrane condoms are not recommended. Instead those made of latex have been found to be effective.* Use of condoms should be supplemented by creams or jelly containing nonxynol 9, a virucidal (kills viruses) agent. The Food and Drug Administration recently stepped up its quality control programs to ensure condom quality. However, the condom is only as safe as the person who uses it, and when there is the occasional failure in condom use, it is more likely failure on the part of the user than the product. Health care officials need to inform their patients on the role of condoms in the prevention of sexually transmitted diseases.

---

* It is very important to remember this. A normal reaction in this situation would be to buy the best condom available. Under normal conditions, the best, and usually the most expensive, condoms are those made from natural membranes. However, in this situation, where AIDS is the primary reason for the purchase of the prophylactic, a good quality latex should be purchased, not one made of natural membrane.

The hesitant and still reluctant cooperation of the media to handle condom advertising has been a barrier in effective AIDS education. Some prominent publications, such as The New York Times, Newsweek, and Time, have agreed to carry condom advertising. These messages have stressed the use of condoms as a disease prevention rather than a means of contraception. While most television stations have resisted requests for condom advertisement, many observers note the irony of blatant sex scenes on day and night time soap operas with virtually no mention of the need to take precautions. Continued education on the proper use of condoms, more aggressive media messages, and accessibility of the product are necessary if prophylactics are to provide significant protection against AIDS.

CHANGING BEHAVIOR

With proper counseling, treatment, education, and rehabilitation, behavior can be altered. Homosexual men must be warned that engaging in sex without condom protection is very risky. Several studies indicate that bisexual and homosexual males have been changing their sexual behavior as a result of the epidemic in an attempt to halt the spread. Heterosexuals need to know that numerous partners increases their risk of infection.

At the same time, those engaged in a long-term, faithful relationship with only one partner need to know that they are at very little risk and have no need to change their behavior. Proper education and prevention programs should promote behavior that does not transmit AIDS.

A MESSAGE FROM THE SURGEON GENERAL

During Spring 1988, the U.S. Surgeon General, C. Everett Koop, sent a copy of the brochure Understanding AIDS to every American household trying to educate the public on AIDS. It discussed, as Dr. Koop observed, issues which many people were not used to discussing openly, but which had to be discussed. Risky sexual behavior by persons of all sexual orientations, the dangers of drugs, and false rumors of "catching" AIDS were all discussed. The Surgeon General recommended responsible behavior and strong values as everyone's personal prevention against AIDS.

Due to the sensitive nature of the material, and the fact that the audience was so vast and diverse, the Administration was expecting numerous calls and letters objecting to the publications. By mid-June the Surgeon General's Office reported that the majority of the calls had been favorable. Many people wanted further explanation and others requested the Spanish-language edition.

EDUCATION AND PREVENTION AMONG SPECIAL GROUPS

Health care workers

On August 21, 1987, the Centers for Disease Control released Recommendation for Prevention of HIV Transmission in Health-Care Settings (MMWR Supplement Vol. 36, No.2S). The CDC emphatically stated that medical histories and examinations are not always reliable indicators of patients with HIV and precaution in handling blood and body fluids should be used consistently with all patients, especially those in emergency-care settings where exposure to blood is increased and the infection status of the patient is often unknown.

Among these precautions are the wearing of gloves, which should be changed after each patient contact when handling bodily fluids, non-intact skin, and for procedures which involve punctures. Hands should be washed immediately after the removal of gloves and if contaminated with blood or blood products. Masks and protective eyewear or face shields are required for procedures which are likely to generate blood droplets or other bodily fluids. Gowns and aprons are necessary for procedures likely to generate splashes of those elements. Although transmittal of HIV through saliva has not been proven, resuscitation bags or other ventilation devises should be made available to avoid the need for mouth-to-mouth resuscitation. Pregnant health care workers are urged to be especially carefully since their infection also puts their unborn children at risk.

All dental workers should wear surgical masks and protective eyewear in addition to gloves. All instruments and apparatus which may have been contaminated by blood, saliva, or gingival fluid should be sterilized. Detailed guidelines are also listed for those who engage in autopsies or morticians' services, dialysis treatment, and laboratory work. (For a discussion of health care workers who have become infected, see Chapter VIII.)

Schools

In a similar release in January 1988, the CDC set forth its recommendations for educating the nation's schoolchildren. In Guidelines for Effective School Health Education To Prevent the Spread of AIDS (MMWR Supplement Vol. 37, No. S-2), guidelines were developed to assist school personnel plan, implement, and evaluate educational efforts to prevent further spread of AIDS and other HIV-related illnesses. While they were intended for school personnel, others who have contact with children, but who are not in school and may therefore, be at even greater risk of becoming infected, should follow these guidelines.

Schools should provide programs and information that will encourage and enable those who have engaged in sexual intercourse to abstain from sexual intercourse until they are ready for a monogamous relationship within a marriage. Those who have not used illicit drugs, should be encouraged to continue not using illicit drugs and those who have used such drugs should be urged to stop. Realizing that despite repeated and well-meaning efforts on the part of those in authority, some young people will continue risky behavior, preventative measures are recommended as a last resort. Young people are urged to refrain from sex with an infected person, to use a latex condom if engaging in sexual intercourse, to not share needles, and to seek counseling and testing if they suspect they are infected.

The principle function of education in the early elementary grades is to allay excessive fears about being infected. Young children are to be told that AIDS causes some adults to get very sick, but commonly children are not affected. AIDS is not transmitted through casual contact, such as touching. Scientists worldwide are working to stop the spread and cure those who have it.

By late elementary school, the children should be exposed to a bit more detail. They are told that AIDS is caused by a virus, a microscopic living organism that can be transmitted from an infected to an uninfected person through a variety of means. AIDS is described as breaking down of the ability to fight off certain infections and diseases. These children should be advised of the scope of the problem and given some detail of the means of transmission: sexual contact, shared needles, and through pregnancy. They are also told that most people with AIDS die within two years after their symptoms appear.

QUESTION: Which of the following steps, if any, have you, yourself, taken or do you plan to take to avoid contracting AIDS? Avoiding elective surgery that would require blood transfusions.

	June 8-14, 1987 (Telephone)			
	Have taken	Have not taken	No opinion	Number of Interviews
NATIONAL	**42%**	**54%**	**4%**	**1,005**
SEX				
Men	41	55	4	505
Women	42	53	5	500
AGE				
18-29 years	44	53	3	231
30-49 years	44	52	4	401
50 & older	38	57	5	370
REGION				
East	40	56	4	255
Midwest	40	57	3	260
South	45	51	4	302
West	41	53	6	188
RACE				
Whites	41	55	4	863
Non-whites	47	49	4	140
Blacks	42	53	5	102
EDUCATION				
College graduates	37	59	4	287
College incomplete	40	58	2	263
High school graduates	43	52	5	331
Not high school grads.	46	48	6	122
POLITICS				
Republicans	38	57	5	307
Democrats	40	56	4	330
Independents	45	52	3	340
HOUSEHOLD INCOME				
$40,000 & over	34	62	4	251
$25,000-$39,999	45	51	4	219
$15,000-$24,999	41	56	3	212
Under $15,000	44	52	4	238
RELIGION				
Protestants	41	54	5	586
Catholics	41	56	3	271

QUESTION: Which of the following steps, if any, have you, yourself, taken or do you plan to take to avoid contracting AIDS? Avoiding the use of restrooms in public facilities.

	June 8-14, 1987 (Telephone)			
	Have taken	Have not taken	No opinion	Number of Interviews
NATIONAL	**28%**	**71%**	**1%**	**1,005**
SEX				
Men	26	73	1	505
Women	30	69	1	500
AGE				
18-29 years	28	72	*	231
30-49 years	25	75	*	401
50 & older	32	67	1	370
REGION				
East	26	74	*	255
Midwest	27	73	*	260
South	35	64	1	302
West	23	76	1	188
RACE				
Whites	26	73	1	863
Non-whites	42	58	*	140
Blacks	44	56	*	102
EDUCATION				
College graduates	16	84	*	287
College incomplete	19	80	*	263
High school graduates	33	66	1	331
Not high school grads.	43	56	1	122
POLITICS				
Republicans	24	76	*	307
Democrats	31	68	1	330
Independents	29	70	1	340
HOUSEHOLD INCOME				
$40,000 & over	18	82	*	251
$25,000-$39,999	22	78	*	219
$15,000-$24,999	24	75	1	212
Under $15,000	42	58	*	238
RELIGION				
Protestants	30	69	1	586
Catholics	26	74	*	271

Source: The Gallup Poll, Princeton, NJ

By junior and senior high, the information is no different from that given to an adult. Older students should be told explicitly of sexual transmission, both in homosexual and heterosexual instances. Risk of infection should be emphasized as well as methods of precaution.

Law Enforcement Officers

Law enforcement officers probably have more contact with persons who are HIV infected or at high risk for infection than any occupation other than health care workers. When they arrive on the scene of an accident, a violent crime, or a domestic incident, they run the risk of contact with blood and other bodily fluids. They have frequent contact with those who are at risk, such as drug addicts and prostitutes. Police officers are often bit, cut, scratched, and attacked while performing their duties.

On August 2, 1987, the National Institute of Justice (NIJ) urged police departments nationwide to develop clear-cut policies for dealing with people infected with the AIDS virus. The NIJ has begun publishing a series of AIDS Bulletins designed to assist those involved in criminal justice to reduce the risk of infection without compromising effective duty performance. Suggestions include, wearing gloves when blood or body fluid contact is likely; avoiding needlesticks; avoiding contact between one's face and hands while on duty, hand washing, and proper disposal of blood and contaminated items. Officers are advised to have suspects empty their own pockets, to use long-handled mirrors for searching hidden areas, to wear protective gloves, to store sharp items in puncture-proof containers, and to use tape instead of staples when packaging evidence. Cities are also urged to make devices available to their officers which make cardiopulmonary resuscitation less risky.

WHAT THE PUBLIC REALLY DOES

For some time now, the public has been bombarded with the ways of preventing AIDS, how to limit or alleviate high risk behavior, and the ways in which AIDS is not transmitted. In June 1987, the Gallup Poll surveyed 1,005 people to determine the methods being taken to avoid infection. Almost three-fourths of those polled claimed to be involved in some sort of preventive measure.

QUESTION: Which of the following steps, if any, have you, yourself, taken or do you plan to take to avoid contracting AIDS? Avoiding elective surgery that would require blood transfusions.

	June 8-14, 1987 (Telephone)			
	Have taken	Have not taken	No opinion	Number of interviews
NATIONAL	**19%**	**73%**	**8%**	**1,005**
SEX				
Men	20	76	4	505
Women	19	71	10	500
AGE				
18-29 years	26	72	2	231
30-49 years	18	77	5	401
50 & older	16	71	13	370
REGION				
East	15	77	8	255
Midwest	15	79	6	260
South	27	64	9	302
West	18	76	6	188
RACE				
Whites	17	75	8	863
Non-whites	34	62	4	140
Blacks	36	58	6	102
EDUCATION				
College graduates	12	86	2	287
College incomplete	18	75	7	263
High school graduates	19	74	7	331
Not high school grads.	29	57	14	122
POLITICS				
Republicans	15	77	8	307
Democrats	23	69	8	330
Independents	19	75	6	340
HOUSEHOLD INCOME				
$40,000 & over	10	84	6	251
$25,000-$39,999	16	80	4	219
$15,000-$24,999	17	76	7	212
Under $15,000	28	62	10	238
RELIGION				
Protestants	20	72	8	586
Catholics	19	76	5	271

Source: The Gallup Poll, Princeton, NJ

QUESTION: Which of the following steps, if any, have you, yourself, taken or do you plan to take to avoid contracting AIDS? Donating your own blood for possible future use.

	June 8-14, 1987 (Telephone)			
	Have taken	Have not taken	No opinion	Number of Interviews
NATIONAL	**42%**	**53%**	**5%**	**1,005**
SEX				
Men	42	54	4	505
Women	42	51	7	500
AGE				
18-29 years	43	56	1	231
30-49 years	46	51	3	401
50 & older	36	53	11	370
REGION				
East	38	58	4	255
Midwest	41	52	7	260
South	41	53	6	302
West	47	48	5	188
RACE				
Whites	42	53	5	863
Non-whites	43	52	5	140
Blacks	44	52	4	102
EDUCATION				
College graduates	43	53	4	287
College incomplete	44	52	4	263
High school graduates	44	52	4	331
Not high school grads.	33	55	12	122
POLITICS				
Republicans	41	53	6	307
Democrats	42	53	5	330
Independents	42	53	5	340
HOUSEHOLD INCOME				
$40,000 & over	41	55	4	251
$25,000-$39,999	47	49	4	219
$15,000-$24,999	41	53	6	212
Under $15,000	38	54	8	238
RELIGION				
Protestants	42	53	5	586
Catholics	44	52	4	271

QUESTION: Which of the following steps, if any, have you, yourself, taken or do you plan to take to avoid contracting AIDS? Not associating with people who you suspect might have AIDS.

	June 8-14, 1987 (Telephone)			
	Have taken	Have not taken	No opinion	Number of Interviews
NATIONAL	**43%**	**49%**	**8%**	**1,005**
SEX				
Men	49	43	8	505
Women	37	55	8	500
AGE				
18-29 years	60	36	4	231
30-49 years	42	48	10	401
50 & older	32	60	8	370
REGION				
East	40	52	8	255
Midwest	45	47	8	260
South	47	46	7	302
West	40	52	8	188
RACE				
Whites	43	49	8	863
Non-whites	44	52	4	140
Blacks	42	53	5	102
EDUCATION				
College graduates	37	55	8	287
College incomplete	41	51	8	263
High school graduates	49	45	6	331
Not high school grads.	40	49	11	122
POLITICS				
Republicans	44	49	7	307
Democrats	45	48	7	330
Independents	40	51	9	340
HOUSEHOLD INCOME				
$40,000 & over	33	59	8	251
$25,000-$39,999	44	47	9	219
$15,000-$24,999	45	50	5	212
Under $15,000	48	45	7	238
RELIGION				
Protestants	43	49	8	586
Catholics	46	49	5	271

Source: The Gallup Poll, Princeton, NJ

Forty-three percent reported that they were not associating with persons they suspected might have AIDS. Sixty percent of those aged 18-29 reported taking this precaution, probably a wise decision for this age group, since the largest proportion of persons with AIDS fall into this group. While associating was not defined, it could well go so far as to mean sexual contact. College graduates and those with higher incomes were least likely to take this precaution.

Preventive Activities

More than two out of five (42 percent) reported that they were avoiding elective surgery that would require blood transfusions and the same proportion were donating their own blood for possible future use. Those aged 50 and older were less likely to bank their own blood, or avoid elective surgery.

Slightly more than one quarter of those polled (28 percent) had stopped using public restrooms as a preventive measure. Blacks, those without high school diplomas, and those with incomes less than $15,000 annually were more likely to take this precaution. In spite of the widespread information that AIDS is not spread this way, there are still many who doubt.

Fortunately, less than 20 percent reported that they had stopped giving blood as a precaution against AIDS. While there are AIDS victims who became infected with AIDS as a result of a contaminated transfusion, AIDS cannot be transmitted by donating blood. The needles used when blood is donated are only used once and discarded. Young people, blacks, residents of the South, and those with low incomes are most likely to avoid donating blood.

CHAPTER XII

LEGAL AND ETHICAL ISSUES

Attempts to control the spread of AIDS have raised numerous legal issues, many of which remain unresolved. To what extent can the government protect the public safety through blood testing and at the same time protect individuals from discrimination? Should physicians tell a third party of the potential harm they face by being intimate with a person with AIDS? Do health care employees have the right to know that they working with a person or body which is HIV infected? Should laboratory workers be told they are handling HIV-infected bodily fluids or tissue? Where does the right to confidentiality end and the right of a person to know begin? Although AIDS is not the first infectious disease to raise these questions, the stigma attached to this disease has weighted the issue down with social and moral questions.

Protecting the Public Health

There are strong legal precedents supporting measures taken to protect the public health. In Jacobson v. Massachusetts, (197 U.S. 643, 1904), the Supreme Court upheld a local government's requirement for compulsory smallpox vaccination where the disease was already present and spreading. The Public Health Service Act (42 U.S.C. Section 264) calls for making and enforcing regulations to prevent the spread of a communicable disease. Public health interests, however, are not necessarily enough to justify any and all legal actions. The courts must first determine the nature of the risk and then examine the methods used to achieve the desired effect to decide if they are the least restrictive alternatives.

Preventing Discrimination

Section 504 of the Rehabilitation Act of 1973, (29 U.S.C. Section 794) prohibits discrimination in any program or activity receiving federal monies against an otherwise qualified person solely on the basis of a handicap. This regulation covers federal executive agencies and the U.S. Postal Service. It is unclear whether Section 504 applies to those persons with AIDS, ARC or a positive HIV antibody test. A broad interpretation would afford persons with AIDS, ARC, or HIV infection some protection against discrimination, but this protection would not extend to private concerns not receiving federal funds, or programs in institutions, corporations, school, etc. which do not receive federal funds.

The U.S. Supreme Court, on March 3, 1987, addressed, in School Board of Nassau County V. Gene H. Arline (55 LW 4245 ,1987), the issue of discrimination and contagious disease. Gene Arline, a school teacher, was fired from her job after three bouts of tuberculosis. She went to court, claiming the school board could not fire her because she was covered under Section 504 of the Rehabilitation Act of 1973. For those following the case, the real issue was not so much tuberculosis, but another infectious and contagious disease, AIDS. Since neither the original language of the law nor congressional intent mentioned or even alluded to consideration of a contagious disease as a handicap, the Court's decision was considered crucial. In a 7-2 decision, the Court ruled that Section 504 does protect persons with contagious diseases from discrimination. In his majority opinion, Justice William Brennan observed that the law was passed "to ensure that handicapped individuals are not denied access to jobs or other benefits because of the prejudiced attitudes or the ignorance of others."

While AIDS was only mentioned in a footnote of the decision, it does establish a precedent for those suffering with the disease by determining that contagious diseases, especially those which lead to physical impairment and dramatically limit major activity, fall under the definition of handicap. The Arline decision does not mean that employers cannot dismiss someone who is incapable of doing the job, or who pose a medical risk of spreading contagious disease. These decisions to dismiss, however, must be based on specific medical evidence that risk does exist and that an alternative work situation for the employee cannot be found.

This Supreme Court decision directly contradicted a U.S. Justice Department interpretation that, while the physical effects of AIDS were covered by Section 504, the ability to transmit the disease, whether real or imagined, was not a handicap, and therefore, was not protected. In other words, if a Justice Department worker feared that a co-worker with AIDS could transmit the disease, the employer could dismiss the employee with AIDS, whether the fear was rational or not. The Arline ruling is also important since many states tend to follow federal practices in their handicap statues.

VOLUNTARY, ROUTINE, OR MANDATORY TESTING AND SCREENING

The Centers for Disease Control (CDC) considers "screening" the offering of a test to a whole population to determine the members' antibody status. "Testing," on the other hand, implies giving a test to an individual based on his or her request or that of a provider.

To further clarify terms, the epidemiologists for the state of Colorado have defined the following three terms for their policy purposes: voluntary, routine, and mandatory testing. Voluntary testing is that which is initiated by the patient's request, without provision from a health care provider. A routine testing is that which physicians are required to do, or which they offer to their patients with the patient's informed consent. The patient has the right to refuse. Mandatory testing is that which is required with the patient having no right of refusal.

Mass Screening

Currently, no state supports routine or mandatory screening of the general population with the exception of donated blood, plasma, blood by-products, donated tissues, organs, or semen. This position has the overwhelming support of health professionals and health agencies and organizations including the Centers for Disease Control (CDC), the Association of State and

Territorial Health Officers (ASTHO) and the American Medical Association (AMA). Several studies have led many authorities to believe that the high cost of finding one seropositive person in the general population is hard to justify when many more true positives may be found by targeted screening or expanded voluntary programs.

Those who favor mandatory mass screening argue that:

1) If everyone gets tested, no one individual or group needs to be stigmatized.

2) The dread of being tested may sharpen a person's sense of vulnerability, especially one who does not consider himself to be at risk.

3) Knowledge of who harbors the infection can help officials control the epidemic and prevent transmission of the virus.

Those who oppose counter with:

1) The fact that it may take up to 14 months for the HIV antibodies to be detected by current testing methods means that a negative antibody result is not a guarantee that the person is free of the AIDS virus. If people are tested too soon, and found to be negative, they may not practice preventive behavior.

2) There is no evidence that people change their intimate behavior due to the results of HIV testing. CDC studies show that the "awareness of HIV antibody status may only have a minor influence on behavior in people who identify themselves as being at risk of HIV infection." (Although other studies have shown that those who did not consider themselves at risk for HIV infection, when found to be antibody positive, changed their behavior to reduce the risk of transmitting to others.)

Blood, Tissue, Organs

Many states have mandated universal screening in the testing of blood, organs, and tissue to protect the supply. At least five states have laws regulating the routine screening of blood and blood products, organs and/or tissues. Some states have regulations regarding testing of potential sperm donors.

In 1985, the American Red Cross, handler of half of the nation's blood supply, issued a "Blood Service Directive" to its affiliates requiring HIV antibody screening. Before the ELISA test was available, however, the Red Cross had opposed testing blood for possible infection. Many physicians, especially those familiar with infectious diseases, were aware that those most at risk for HIV infection - homosexual/bisexual men, IV drug abusers, and hemophiliacs, were also those most likely to have hepatitis B, for which there was a test. The reluctance and refusal of blood banks to test for hepatitis B, the only test available for a time, helped to spread the epidemic through infected blood. The Food and Drug Administration (FDA), whose job it is to safeguard the nations' blood supply, did not force the testing on the blood banks at that time, but since 1986 has had new regulations pending regarding the screening of all blood and blood products. While no formal national legislation exists, it is now standard practice to screen blood and blood products.

AIDS

STATES THAT ROUTINELY SCREEN PRISONERS AND PROSTITUTES FOR HIV ANTIBODIES

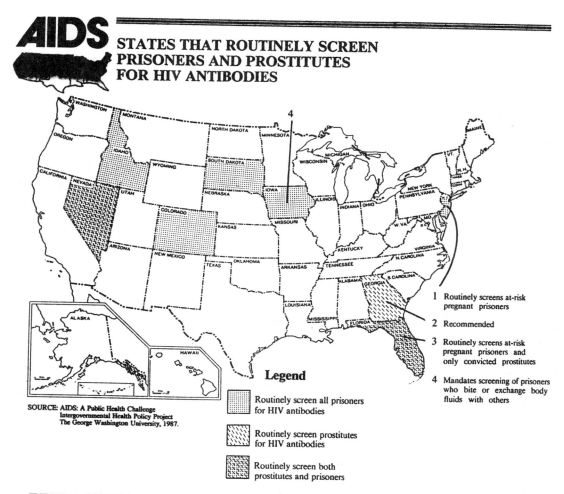

1 Routinely screens at-risk pregnant prisoners

2 Recommended

3 Routinely screens at-risk pregnant prisoners and only convicted prostitutes

4 Mandates screening of prisoners who bite or exchange body fluids with others

Legend

▨ Routinely screen all prisoners for HIV antibodies

▨ Routinely screen prostitutes for HIV antibodies

▨ Routinely screen both prostitutes and prisoners

SOURCE: AIDS: A Public Health Challenge
Intergovernmental Health Policy Project
The George Washington University, 1987.

AIDS

STATES THAT CONSIDERED PREMARITAL TESTING FOR HIV OR STDs IN 1986

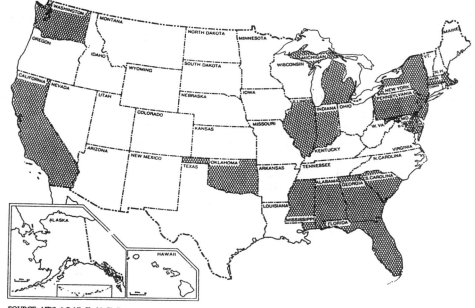

SOURCE: AIDS: A Public Health Challenge
Intergovernmental Health Policy Project
The George Washington University, 1987.

Screening High-Risk Population Groups

In March 1986, the CDC recommended that HIV antibody testing be routinely offered to persons who practice high risk behavior whenever they visited STD (sexually transmitted diseases) clinics, clinics for IV drug abuse, family planning clinics, or clinics providing health care to prostitutes. By May 1987, the CDC, in "Recommended Additional Guidelines for HIV Antibody Counseling and Testing in the Prevention of HIV Infection and AIDS," expanded the earlier guidelines and set standards and priorities for the number of groups and conditions where testing should be routinely offered and encouraged by those providing health care. The consensus of the more than 500 experts and interested parties who attended the conference which drafted these recommendations was that mass or mandatory screening would not be as cost-effective as significantly expanding opportunities for voluntary testing in high-risk areas and among high-risk groups.

The groups and situations CDC deems suitable for routinely offering HIV antibody testing are: 1) those being treated for STD; 2) persons being treated for IV drug use (as well as their sexual or drug-using partners); 3) persons who consider themselves at risk (e.g. those with multiple sex partners over the last five to seven years); 4) high-risk women of child-bearing age (either they practice high-risk behavior or their partners do); 5) women of childbearing age who live in areas with high rates of HIV infection; 6) persons with tuberculosis and selected patients who received blood or blood-product transfusions between 1978 and mid-1985.

In August 1987, the Public Health Service (PHS) issued final recommendations for routine testing HIV antibody testing among these groups and also included prostitutes. As mentioned earlier, "routine" means that the patient can refuse the test. The PHS further urged prison systems to pursue methods of testing inmates and state and local governments to consider routine or mandatory pre-marital testing.

Screening Prisoners

In May 1987 the federal prison system instituted an initial screening program which tested all incoming sentenced inmates; screened all inmates who initially tested negative every six months; and screened all inmates within 60 days prior to release to a halfway house or the community.

Screening at the state level remains a volatile issue. Several states, including Colorado and Connecticut, have questioned the validity of screening all prisoners. Their concern stems from several factors. 1) Since the state is responsible for the health and welfare of all inmates within its jurisdictions, if seropositive prisoners are paroled or released, what becomes of the state's responsibility to all its citizens. 2) The incidence of persons with HIV infection in correctional systems seems to be higher than the general population because the people most likely to be in prison are those with demographic and behavioral characteristics closely associated with AIDS (i.e., young adult males and IV drug users). Screening in state prisons has shown a seropositive rate ranging from 0.2 to 2.5 percent, compared with an incidence of 0.01 percent in the general blood donor population. 3) Although homosexual behavior is prohibited, it is common and difficult to control in institutional situations. 4) IV drug use, like homosexual behavior, is prohibited, but still occurs.

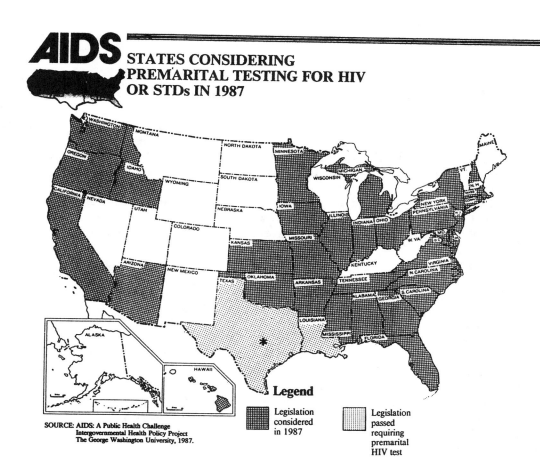

AIDS STATES CONSIDERING PREMARITAL TESTING FOR HIV OR STDs IN 1987

Legend

Legislation considered in 1987

Legislation passed requiring premarital HIV test

* Requires premarital testing when HIV seroprevalence rate = 0.83%

SOURCE: AIDS: A Public Health Challenge
Intergovernmental Health Policy Project
The George Washington University, 1987.

AIDS STATES THAT HAVE REPEALED PREMARITAL TESTING REQUIREMENTS FOR STDs

SOURCE: AIDS: A Public Health Challenge
Intergovernmental Health Policy Project
The George Washington University, 1987.

Screening Prostitutes

Data from Africa, which has a much higher incidence of heterosexual transmission than the U.S., suggests that prostitutes have become an important factor in spreading the AIDS virus on that continent. Because prostitutes have numerous sex partners and are frequently IV drug users, they can be considered high-risk. Research on prostitutes in the U.S. is limited, and it is uncertain what part they play in increasing heterosexual cases.

Nevada is the only state which allows counties the right to make prostitution legal, and therefore the only state which requires routine health exams and testing for HIV antibody among registered prostitutes. According to state officials, only 4 out of 3,000 prostitutes, or about 0.1 percent have tested positive for HIV antibody.

Several other states, which do not have legalized prostitution, have attempted to test those engaged in prostitution. Michigan has proposed a law requiring testing for those arrested for prostitution or solicitation. If found to be HIV positive, the information would be passed on to the judge who would base the conditions for their release pending trial on that information. Similar proposed bills in California, Hawaii, Illinois, North Carolina, and Oklahoma failed to pass. In Florida, anyone arrested for prostitution can request screening for a transmissible disease. If convicted of prostitution, they are required to undergo screening for STD. A Georgia Task Force has recommended that all convicted prostitutes be tested for HIV antibodies, and that education programs should complement the program.

Premarital Screening

In May 1987, President Reagan urged states to consider premarital testing. While more than half of the states have introduced bills over the past several years, only Illinois, Louisiana and Texas have passed laws mandating premarital screening. The Texas law, however, will be implemented only if the seroprevalence rate among the general population increases from the current 0.1 percent to 0.83 percent. This "conditional" legislation characterizes the ambivalence surrounding the question of premarital screening and its cost-effectiveness.

In fact, by April 1988, both Illinois and Louisiana had repealed their laws. The repeal in Louisiana was a unanimous decision of the legislature which characterized the law as an "expensive flop." Hundreds of young couples fled to surrounding states to marry because of the testing for which some physicians and laboratories charged as much as $200.00. Physicians reported that those taking the tests were not in high-risk groups. Illinois reported problems early in its program because many couples were unable to pay the $70 charged for the test. The decision to repeal in Illinois was not as unanimous as that in Louisiana and opposition is expected to continue.

PUBLIC OPINIONS ABOUT TESTING

In June 1987, the Gallup Poll found that the public favors testing a variety of groups in this country to determine the extent of HIV infection. Nine of every ten Americans polled supported testing immigrants who applied for permanent residence in the U.S. Almost that many (88 percent) favored testing federal prison inmates, while eight of ten supported testing those who applied for marriage licenses. Two-thirds of those polled would like to see foreign

STATE STRATEGIES TO
STRENGTHEN CONFIDENTIALITY OF MEDICAL RECORDS

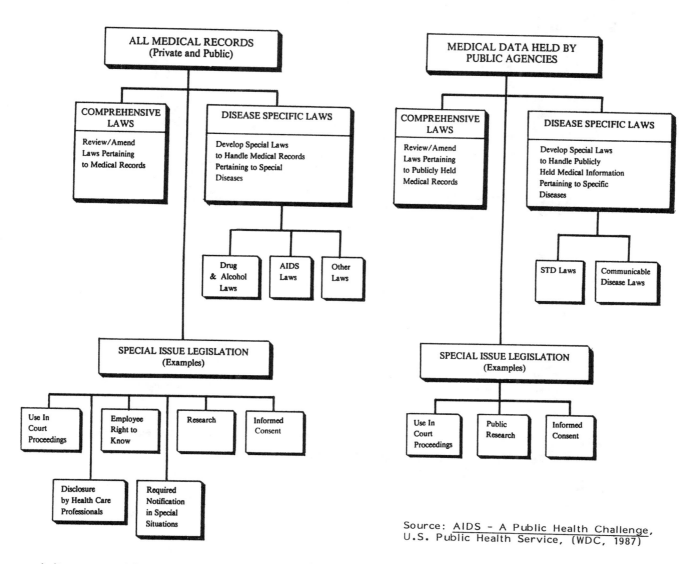

Source: AIDS - A Public Health Challenge, U.S. Public Health Service, (WDC, 1987)

visitors to this country tested. A little more than half of those polled believed that the entire population should be tested. Respondents who were college graduates opposed universal testing by a ratio of 3-to-2, while those who had not graduated high school favored such testing by almost 2-to-1.

STATE LAWS AND CONFIDENTIALITY

The assurance that a physician will not disclose confidential information allows patients the freedom to discuss sensitive issues such as drug use and sexuality. It promotes a sense of dignity and privacy. The professional guidelines for confidentiality are as old as the Hippocratic Oath and as recent as the recommendation from the American College of Physicians which states "the identity of a person diagnosed with HIV-infection should be limited to the greatest extent possible without sacrificing the protection of the public health." However, there are no guidelines specifying which situations endanger the public health and when doctors are responsible for disclosing information. At its July 1988 convention, the American Medical Association (AMA) ruled that physicians could disclose information regarding HIV infection to a patient's sexual partner, if the patient refused to do so.

AIDS STATES THAT PASSED LAWS REGARDING DISCLOSURE

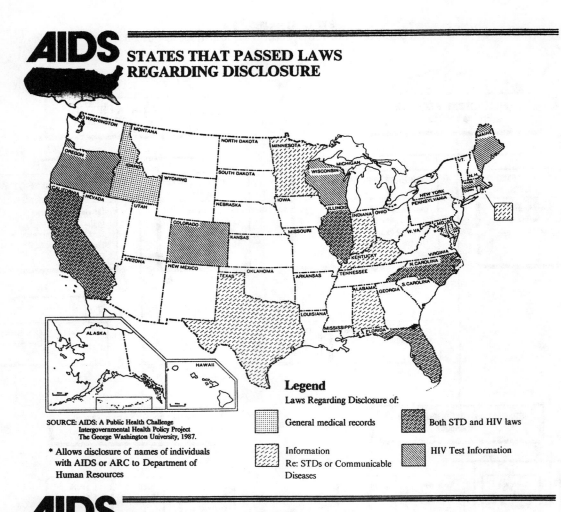

SOURCE: AIDS: A Public Health Challenge
Intergovernmental Health Policy Project
The George Washington University, 1987.

* Allows disclosure of names of individuals
with AIDS or ARC to Department of
Human Resources

Legend

Laws Regarding Disclosure of:

General medical records

Information
Re: STDs or Communicable
Diseases

Both STD and HIV laws

HIV Test Information

AIDS STATES WITH LAWS RELATING TO PENALTIES FOR UNAUTHORIZED DISCLOSURE

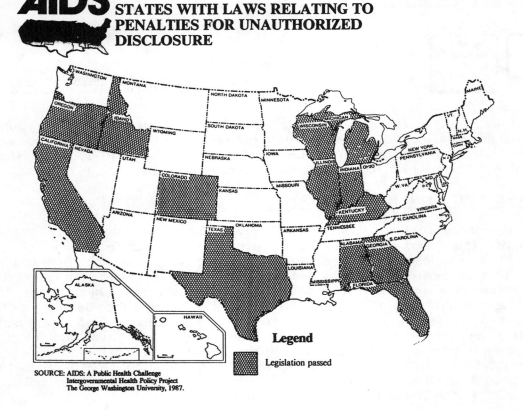

Legend

Legislation passed

SOURCE: AIDS: A Public Health Challenge
Intergovernmental Health Policy Project
The George Washington University, 1987.

Some physicians wear two hats. Those employed by corporations, schools, unions, and the military have an obligation to the employer (the institution), as well as to the individual patient. CDC guidelines point out to those in public health that unauthorized disclosure of personal information may discourage the use of counseling and testing facilities as well as cause the possibility of inappropriate discrimination.

Many states have statutes dealing with the confidentiality of both public and private medical records, the required reporting of personal health information for public health purposes, and the confidentiality of public health information. However, states also have exemptions to physician-patient confidentiality for law-enforcement purposes, such as reporting gunshot wounds, child abuse, dog bites, and similar situations.

States have chosen a wide variety of strategies for addressing confidentiality. Not many states have adopted policies which cover handling private and public medical records. Some states have simply confined their interpretation of confidentiality to safeguarding medical records. Others have focused solely on public health data because of the concern about the handling of information that identifies HIV-infected individuals by health officials. Some states have limited the disclosure of public health records to subpoena situations or disclosure in closed court proceedings. Others have relied on existing laws relating to sexually transmitted or communicable diseases to determine confidentiality as it pertains to AIDS.

Some states require reporting to health authorities all those known to be HIV infected; other states ask for the reporting of only those HIV-infected persons who also have developed AIDS; other states require health officials to track AIDS sufferers, while others only ask that state health officials keep a record of their names. Some states keep only anonymous reports.

THE QUESTION OF QUARANTINE

Recent events such as the barring from school and the burning of the home of three small Arcadia, FL brothers, all hemophiliacs, and all HIV-infected as a result of contaminated blood products, illustrates how deep the fear of AIDS is among the American people and how unconvinced they are that casual contact with people with AIDS is as safe as some officials are claiming. Quarantine is an emotionally charged word, bringing up images of roundups, leper colonies, and concentration camps. Conservative spokesmen such as Senator Jesse Helms (R-NC) and former presidential candidate Pat Robertson have spoken in favor of quarantine, but have offered no specifics.

In dictatorships such as Cuba, Fidel Castro is free to quarantine over 100 people with the AIDS virus on a farm near Havana. Rounding up the estimated 1.5 million AIDS carriers in this country, would be unconstitutional, and, many health experts feel, unnecessary. Those opposed to quarantines think AIDS is unlike other infectious diseases in that it is not easily spread and those who are infected remain that way for life. Therefore, since there is no cure, to quarantine these carriers would mean a life sentence.

Since 1985, at least nine states have either amended or passed quarantine laws authorizing health officials to isolate those individuals with AIDS who endanger other people's health. As the laws about reporting and confidentiality, the laws on quarantine vary considerably. For example, Colorado's new law applies only to HIV infection and AIDS and calls for up to three months of iso-

QUESTION: In your opinion, which of the following groups of people, if any, should be tested for AIDS?: Visitors from foreign countries?

June 8-14, 1987 (Telephone)

	Should	Should not	No opinion	Number of Interviews
NATIONAL	66%	30%	4%	1,005
SEX				
Men	62	34	4	505
Women	69	26	5	500
AGE				
18-29 years	68	32	*	231
30-49 years	62	34	4	401
50 & older	69	25	6	370
REGION				
East	67	28	5	255
Midwest	62	35	3	260
South	70	26	4	302
West	62	32	6	188
RACE				
Whites	64	31	5	863
Non-whites	77	21	2	140
Blacks	76	22	2	102
EDUCATION				
College graduates	49	46	5	287
College incomplete	62	35	3	263
High school graduates	71	25	4	331
Not high school grads.	78	16	6	122
POLITICS				
Republicans	60	35	5	307
Democrats	73	24	3	330
Independents	61	35	4	340
HOUSEHOLD INCOME				
$40,000 & over	52	44	4	251
$25,000-$39,999	61	34	5	219
$15,000-$24,999	69	29	2	212
Under $15,000	76	20	4	238
RELIGION				
Protestants	66	29	5	586
Catholics	68	29	3	271

Source: The Gallup Poll, Princeton, NJ

QUESTION: In your opinion, which of the following groups of people, if any, should be tested for AIDS?: All American citizens?

June 8-14, 1987 (Telephone)

	Should	Should not	No opinion	Number of Interviews
NATIONAL	52%	45%	3%	1,005
SEX				
Men	51	46	3	505
Women	53	44	3	500
AGE				
18-29 years	50	49	1	231
30-49 years	49	50	1	401
50 & older	57	39	4	370
REGION				
East	50	48	2	255
Midwest	49	47	4	260
South	60	38	2	302
West	48	49	3	188
RACE				
Whites	52	46	2	863
Non-whites	55	42	3	140
Blacks	57	42	1	102
EDUCATION				
College graduates	39	58	3	287
College incomplete	48	49	3	263
High school graduates	56	42	2	331
Not high school grads.	64	34	2	122
POLITICS				
Republicans	51	46	3	307
Democrats	55	42	3	330
Independents	48	50	2	340
HOUSEHOLD INCOME				
$40,000 & over	42	54	4	251
$25,000-$39,999	47	51	2	219
$15,000-$24,999	51	46	3	212
Under $15,000	61	37	2	238
RELIGION				
Protestants	52	45	3	586
Catholics	52	46	2	271

QUESTION: In your opinion, which of the following groups of people, if any, should be tested for AIDS?: Inmates of federal prisons.

June 8-14, 1987 (Telephone)

	Should	Should not	No opinion	Number of Interviews
NATIONAL	**88%**	**10%**	**2%**	**1,005**
SEX				
Men	88	11	1	505
Women	88	10	2	500
AGE				
18-29 years	87	11	1	231
30-49 years	85	14	1	401
50 & older	91	5	4	370
REGION				
East	86	12	2	255
Midwest	85	12	3	260
South	91	7	2	302
West	88	11	1	188
RACE				
Whites	88	10	2	863
Non-whites	90	9	1	140
Blacks	89	10	1	102
EDUCATION				
College graduates	82	15	3	287
College incomplete	90	9	1	263
High school graduates	87	11	2	331
Not high school grads.	93	5	2	122
POLITICS				
Republicans	92	6	2	307
Democrats	85	14	1	330
Independents	87	11	2	340
HOUSEHOLD INCOME				
$40,000 & over	86	12	2	251
$25,000-$39,999	91	8	1	219
$15,000-$24,999	86	12	2	212
Under $15,000	89	8	3	238
RELIGION				
Protestants	88	10	2	586
Catholics	89	9	2	271

Source: The Gallup Poll, Princeton, NJ

QUESTION: In your opinion, which of the following groups of people, if any, should be tested for AIDS?: Couples applying for marriage licenses.

June 8-14, 1987 (Telephone)

	Should	Should not	No opinion	Number of Interviews
NATIONAL	**80%**	**18%**	**2%**	**1,005**
SEX				
Men	79	18	3	505
Women	81	18	1	500
AGE				
18-29 years	71	27	2	231
30-49 years	79	20	1	401
50 & older	87	10	3	370
REGION				
East	83	16	1	255
Midwest	78	20	2	260
South	82	16	2	302
West	76	21	3	188
RACE				
Whites	81	17	2	863
Non-whites	76	22	2	140
Blacks	73	25	2	102
EDUCATION				
College graduates	78	21	1	287
College incomplete	76	21	3	263
High school graduates	81	17	2	331
Not high school grads.	86	13	1	122
POLITICS				
Republicans	83	15	2	307
Democrats	78	20	2	330
Independents	78	20	2	340
HOUSEHOLD INCOME				
$40,000 & over	79	18	3	251
$25,000-$39,999	83	16	1	219
$15,000-$24,999	77	20	3	212
Under $15,000	83	16	1	238
RELIGION				
Protestants	80	18	2	586
Catholics	81	18	1	271

QUESTION: In your opinion, which of the following groups of people, if any, should be tested for AIDS?: Immigrants applying for permanent residence in the U.S.

June 8-14, 1987 (Telephone)

	Should	Should not	No opinion	Number of Interviews
NATIONAL	90%	9%	1%	1,005
SEX				
Men	90	9	1	505
Women	90	9	1	500
AGE				
18-29 years	88	12	•	231
30-49 years	88	10	2	401
50 & older	93	6	1	370
REGION				
East	90	10	•	255
Midwest	87	12	1	260
South	92	6	2	302
West	90	9	1	188
EDUCATION				
College graduates	86	13	1	287
College incomplete	91	7	2	263
High school graduates	89	10	1	331
Not high school grads.	94	5	1	122
RACE				
Whites	90	9	1	863
Non-whites	88	12	•	140
Blacks	87	13	•	102
POLITICS				
Republicans	92	6	2	307
Democrats	89	10	1	330
Independents	88	12	•	340
HOUSEHOLD INCOME				
$40,000 & over	87	11	2	251
$25,000-$39,999	91	8	1	219
$15,000-$24,999	88	11	1	212
Under $15,000	93	6	1	238
RELIGION				
Protestants	91	8	1	586
Catholics	89	10	1	271

Source: The Gallup Poll, Princeton, NJ

QUESTION: In your opinion, which of the following groups of people, if any, should be tested for AIDS?: Members of the armed forces.

June 8-14, 1987 (Telephone)

	Should	Should not	No opinion	Number of Interviews
NATIONAL	83%	14%	3%	1,005
SEX				
Men	81	16	3	505
Women	84	13	3	500
AGE				
18-29 years	80	19	1	231
30-49 years	79	18	3	401
50 & older	89	7	4	370
REGION				
East	81	15	4	255
Midwest	78	19	3	260
South	88	9	3	302
West	85	14	1	188
EDUCATION				
College graduates	79	18	3	287
College incomplete	81	17	2	263
High school graduates	84	12	4	331
Not high school grads.	88	9	3	122
RACE				
Whites	83	13	4	863
Non-whites	80	18	2	140
Blacks	80	18	2	102
POLITICS				
Republicans	85	10	5	307
Democrats	84	14	2	330
Independents	80	18	2	340
HOUSEHOLD INCOME				
$40,000 & over	79	17	4	251
$25,000-$39,999	83	13	4	219
$15,000-$24,999	83	15	2	212
Under $15,000	87	11	2	238
RELIGION				
Protestants	84	13	3	586
Catholics	85	11	4	271

lation. Minnesota has a law with a six-month limit and covers all communicable diseases. North Carolina's law gives health officials the right to limit the "freedom of movement or action" of those known to have a communicable disease. The new laws, unlike many of the older laws, consider quarantining a last resort after all other restrictive methods have failed.

The few quarantine orders that have been implemented, were issued primarily against male and female prostitutes. Most were lifted before a court battle could settle any constitutional issues. Even the states which allow isolation have been reluctant to implement it. Many attorneys and public health officials believe that the old laws regulating quarantined individuals would not be found constitutional today if applied to AIDS cases in light of the Supreme Court's expanded view of due process, which protects persons from arbitrary actions by states.

THE QUESTION OF CRIME

At least five states (LA, NV, AL, FL, ID) have passed new laws which make knowingly transmitting AIDS a crime under some circumstances. The Alabama law affects those who conduct themselves "in a manner likely to transmit" a sexually transmitted disease. The Nevada law is more specific: charges of attempted murder could be filed against prostitutes who continue in their business after learning they are HIV infected. Some states have existing laws which deal with transmission of a venereal disease, but not all states consider AIDS a venereal disease.

CAN HEALTH CARE WORKERS SAY "NO"?

Several cases have occurred among health care workers, particularly doctors and nurses, who, fearing for their own safety and that of their families, have refused to treat an AIDS-infected person or someone they suspect to be infected. Professional associations have just begun to address the issue of the threat of HIV infection to their members as well as the members' responsibility, if any, to treat those infected. There are some both within and outside the health care professions who believe that physicians are not obligated to expose themselves to even small risks. The exceptions are those physicians who work in hospital emergency rooms or in public hospitals. Those who disagree say that all physicians are required to assume some risk.

In 1987, the American Medical Association (AMA), in its Report of the Council on Ethical and Judicial Affairs: Ethical Issues Involved in the Growing AIDS Crisis (Chicago, 1987), stated that a "physician may not ethically refuse to treat a patient whose condition is within the physician's current realm of competence" simply because the patient has AIDS or has tested seropositive for the AIDS virus." (p.4) The American Nurses' Association has indicated that "Nursing is resolute in its perspective that care should be delivered without prejudice, and it makes no allowance for use of the patient's personal attributes or socioeconomic status or the nature of the health problems as grounds for discrimination." (American Nurses' Association, Committee on Ethics; Statement regarding risk versus responsibility in providing nursing care. (p. 1) (Kansas City, 1986)) There have been no recorded instances of a health care professional losing his or her license to practice by refusing to treat AIDS patients, nor, at this time, are any expected.

CHAPTER XIII

WHAT WE KNOW AND WHAT WE FEEL

In spite of the fact that the American public is bombarded with information about acquired immune deficiency syndrome (AIDS), the methods of transmission and prevention, the cost in lives and dollars, and the identification of high risk factors and groups, there is still a sizable gap between what people know about the disease and how we feel about it and the people who have fallen victim to it.

A PUBLIC HEALTH SERVICE STUDY

The National Center for Health Statistics, of the U.S. Public Health Service, questioned the adult population on their knowledge and attitudes about AIDS in the National Health Interview Survey (NHIS) in August 1987 and the five subsequent months. The most recent findings were published in AIDS Knowledge and Attitudes for December 1987: Provisional Data From the National Health Interview Survey (Hyattsville, MD, May 16, 1988). In most cases, the questions were asked verbatim to those reproduced in the accompanying tables, although a few questions or categories were rephrased or combined. Refusals or nonresponses were excluded from the calculation estimates, but "don't know" responses were included. The accompanying graphs illustrate the changes in attitudes and knowledge in the five months of the survey, due largely, no doubt to increased education.

Awareness of AIDS

Not surprisingly, considering the enormity of the problem and the continued discussion of patients and risks, virtually everyone (more than 99 percent) had heard of AIDS. Three-fourths of the adults had last seen, heard, or read something on the subject of AIDS within 3 days of the NHIS interview. Adults in the 30-49 age group (incidentally, the ages of many AIDS victims) had the most recent knowledge of AIDs, as did whites and married persons.

Self-perceived Knowledge

Only 22 percent of those interviewed felt that, compared to most people, they knew a lot about AIDS; 40 percent believed they knew some; 27 percent thought they knew a little; and 11 percent felt they knew nothing. Persons over age 50 (22 percent) and blacks (17 percent) were far more likely to indicate they knew nothing about the disease than the rest of the population. In fact, blacks were almost twice as likely as whites (10 percent) to say they knew nothing about AIDS.

General Knowledge

When questioned about the definite or probable truth of selected statements about AIDS, the depth of knowledge varied. An overwhelming majority (92 percent) were certain AIDS led to death, while another 7 percent were somewhat less certain. No one disagreed. A somewhat smaller majority (86 percent) knew there was definite truth to the statement that there is no cure. About 82 percent of the adults knew that AIDS can be sexually transmitted, while another 14 percent thought it was probably true. Over three-quarters (77 percent) of the adults in this country definitely think that a pregnant woman who has the AIDS virus can pass it on to her child and almost that many (72 percent) think that AIDS cripples the body's abilities to fight disease.

Knowledge about the nature of AIDS and its viral make-up is less certain. Less than half (47 percent) of American adults definitely believe that a virus causes AIDS, another 27 percent believe with less certainty. More than half of the adults were certain that a person could be infected with the AIDS virus, but not have the disease AIDS, and slightly more than half that many (24 percent) thought that was probably true. The least amount of certainty was found when respondents were faced with statements about the specific ways AIDS can effect it victims. For example, only one-quarter (26 percent) of the respondents were certain that AIDS can damage the brain. Overall, those in the 50 years and above age group, consistent with their self-assessment about their relative lack of knowledge about the disease, had the lowest level of general information.

Transmission of the Virus

Most Americans know how the AIDS virus is most likely transmitted. Ninety-four percent of adults said it was very likely that AIDS could be transmitted sexually and 93 percent thought it was very likely transmitted by sharing drug-use needles with a person who had AIDS. At the same time, the level of misinformation about transmissions is also relatively high. Thirty-four percent of those interviewed felt there was some likelihood that AIDS could be transmitted from donating blood, while 28 percent believed that working near someone with AIDS was a possible source of transmission. Sharing eating utensils with someone with AIDS was considered risky by over half (53 percent); using toilet facilities by 39 percent; and being bitten by mosquitoes and other insects by 42 percent. Black respondents were considerably more likely than their white counterparts to fear an AIDS infection from various types of casual contact.

Testing for the Virus

Generally, seven out of ten Americans had heard about the blood test for AIDS, primarily those in the 30-49 age group (81 percent). Those ages 50 and over were least likely to have heard of it (59 percent). Unfortunately, while there is widespread awareness of the blood test, many adults misunderstand the purpose. Forty percent (more than half of those who had heard of the test) erroneously believed the test tells if the person has AIDS, when it actually tests for the presence of the AIDS virus. A person can be infected with the AIDS virus, and still not have the disease, AIDS. A diagnosis and the presence of other disorders are needed to establish the presence of the AIDS disease.

Less than one out 10 reported having their blood tested for the AIDS virus. Of this proportion, 2 percent volunteered that they had been tested

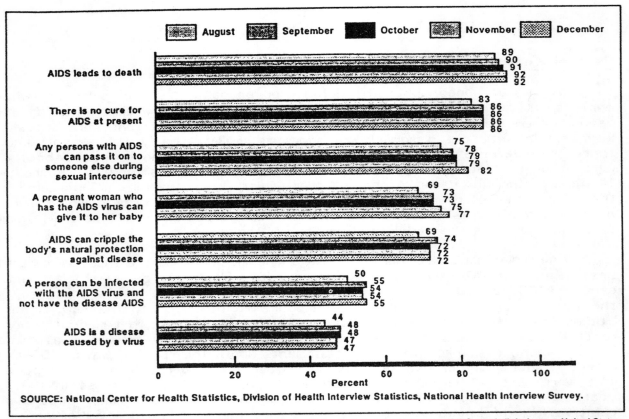

SOURCE: National Center for Health Statistics, Division of Health Interview Statistics, National Health Interview Survey.

Estimated percent of adults 18 years of age and over who think selected statements about AIDS are definitely true: United States, August-December 1987

because of a blood transfusion or donation. Interestingly, about 12 percent of the respondents reported having giving blood since January 1985, which is the approximate date that routine testing of donated blood began.

Who Is At Risk?

Most Americans feel they and the people that they know are at little or no risk of AIDS virus infection. More than 9 out 10 felt there was no chance (63 percent) or a low chance (29 percent) that they would get AIDS. Six out of 10 thought the chance of someone they know getting AIDS was low (36 percent) or nonexistent (26 percent). Seven percent of Americans over age 18 reported personally knowing someone with the AIDS virus. The odds are that proportion will increase in the next decade.

The large proportion of those who felt they and others they knew were not at high risk is interesting when considering the relatively high number of those who believed the AIDS virus could be casually transmitted. Either they may not believe they have contact with those in high risk groups who could transmit the virus to them, or they are being optimistic in their perception of their risk.

Prevention, Discussion, and Education

About 90 percent of those interviewed recognized that celibacy and re-stricting sexual activity to a monogamous relationship with someone free of the AIDS virus are very effective ways of avoiding infection. Use of condoms was considered very effective by 36 percent, while another 47 percent considered this method somewhat effective. More than half of Americans thought using a diaphragm was an ineffective way to avoid infection the of AIDS virus, as was the use of spermicides.

112

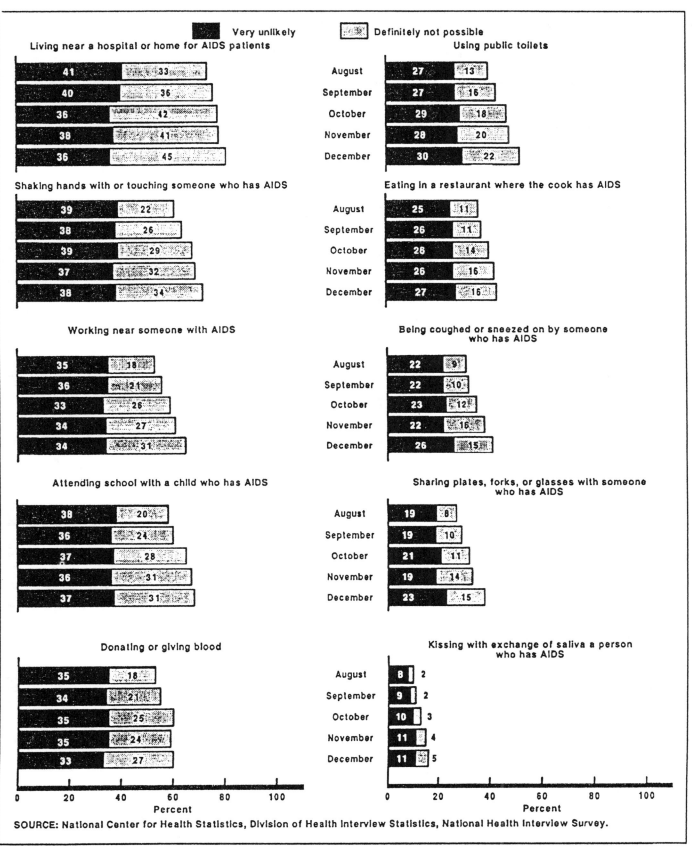

Legend: ■ Very unlikely   ▨ Definitely not possible

Living near a hospital or home for AIDS patients

	Very unlikely	Definitely not possible
	41	33
	40	36
	36	42
	38	41
	36	45

Shaking hands with or touching someone who has AIDS

	Very unlikely	Definitely not possible
	39	22
	38	26
	39	29
	37	32
	38	34

Working near someone with AIDS

	Very unlikely	Definitely not possible
	35	18
	36	21
	33	26
	34	27
	34	31

Attending school with a child who has AIDS

	Very unlikely	Definitely not possible
	38	20
	36	24
	37	28
	36	31
	37	31

Donating or giving blood

	Very unlikely	Definitely not possible
	35	18
	34	21
	35	25
	35	24
	33	27

Using public toilets

Month	Very unlikely	Definitely not possible
August	27	13
September	27	16
October	29	18
November	28	20
December	30	22

Eating in a restaurant where the cook has AIDS

Month	Very unlikely	Definitely not possible
August	25	11
September	26	11
October	28	14
November	26	16
December	27	16

Being coughed or sneezed on by someone who has AIDS

Month	Very unlikely	Definitely not possible
August	22	9
September	22	10
October	23	12
November	22	16
December	26	15

Sharing plates, forks, or glasses with someone who has AIDS

Month	Very unlikely	Definitely not possible
August	19	8
September	19	10
October	21	11
November	19	14
December	23	15

Kissing with exchange of saliva a person who has AIDS

Month	Very unlikely	Definitely not possible
August	8	2
September	9	2
October	10	3
November	11	4
December	11	5

SOURCE: National Center for Health Statistics, Division of Health Interview Statistics, National Health Interview Survey.

Estimated percent of adults 18 years of age and over considering it very unlikely or definitely not possible to transmit the AIDS virus in selected ways: United States, August-December 1987

Provisional estimates of the percent of persons 18 years of age and over with selected AIDS knowledge and attitudes from the 1987 National Health Interview Survey, by selected characteristics: United States, December 1987

[Data are based on household interviews of the civilian noninstitutionalized population. The survey design, general qualifications, and information on the reliability of the estimates are given in technical notes]

AIDS knowledge or attitude	Total	Age			Sex		Race		Education		
		18-29 years	30-49 years	50 years and over	Male	Female	White	Black	Less than 12 years	12 years	More than 12 years
					Percent distribution[1]						
Total...........................	100	100	100	100	100	100	100	100	100	100	100
1. Have you ever heard of AIDS? When was the last time you saw, heard, or read something about AIDS?											
0-3 days ago.............................	72	64	73	78	75	70	74	63	68	71	76
4-7 days ago.............................	15	19	15	13	14	17	15	17	15	16	15
8-14 days ago...........................	4	6	3	2	4	3	3	5	5	3	3
15-31 days ago..........................	4	6	5	2	3	5	4	6	4	5	4
More than 31 days ago...................	2	4	2	1	2	3	1	6	3	3	1
Never heard of AIDS....................	–	–	–	–	–	–	–	–	–	–	–
Don't know..............................	2	2	1	3	2	2	2	3	5	2	1
2. Compared to most people, how much would you say you know about AIDS?											
A lot	22	22	28	15	23	21	23	14	8	17	35
Some	40	46	43	33	38	42	41	32	24	44	45
Little	27	28	23	30	28	26	25	35	38	30	17
Nothing	11	4	5	22	12	10	10	18	30	8	2
Don't know..............................	0	–	0	–	0	–	0	–	–	0	0
3a. AIDS is a disease caused by a virus.											
Definitely true...........................	47	57	54	33	51	44	48	45	34	46	56
Probably true............................	27	28	26	26	26	27	26	27	25	27	27
Probably false...........................	4	4	3	6	4	5	5	4	5	5	3
Definitely false..........................	5	4	5	7	4	6	5	5	5	7	4
Don't know..............................	16	8	11	28	15	18	16	19	31	14	10
3b. AIDS can cripple the body's natural protection against disease.											
Definitely true...........................	72	77	79	60	73	71	74	57	49	72	84
Probably true............................	18	17	15	23	18	19	17	24	25	20	13
Probably false...........................	1	1	1	1	1	1	1	2	2	1	1
Definitely false..........................	1	1	1	1	1	1	1	2	2	1	0
Don't know..............................	8	5	5	14	7	9	7	16	22	6	2
3c. AIDS is especially common in older people.											
Definitely true	0	0	0	1	0	0	0	1	1	0	0
Probably true............................	1	1	1	1	1	1	1	2	2	1	1
Probably false...........................	18	20	17	18	18	18	18	17	17	18	18
Definitely false..........................	73	71	77	70	72	74	74	67	63	75	77
Don't know..............................	8	7	5	11	8	7	7	13	17	6	4
3d. The AIDS virus can damage the brain.											
Definitely true...........................	26	22	27	27	27	25	25	32	25	25	26
Probably true............................	32	33	31	32	32	32	32	32	31	33	32
Probably false...........................	8	9	9	6	8	8	9	6	4	8	11
Definitely false..........................	7	10	8	4	8	6	7	3	5	7	8
Don't know..............................	27	26	25	31	25	29	27	27	36	27	22
3e. AIDS usually leads to heart disease.											
Definitely true	7	6	7	8	7	7	7	13	9	7	6
Probably true............................	22	22	22	23	23	22	22	25	22	23	22
Probably false...........................	18	19	20	13	18	17	19	9	9	17	23
Definitely false..........................	14	16	18	9	16	13	15	10	9	13	18
Don't know..............................	38	36	33	47	36	41	38	43	50	39	31
3f. AIDS leads to death.											
Definitely true	92	93	93	89	92	92	92	92	88	93	93
Probably true............................	7	6	6	8	7	6	7	6	7	6	7
Probably false...........................	0	0	0	0	0	0	0	–	0	0	0
Definitely false..........................	0	0	0	0	0	0	0	–	0	0	0
Don't know..............................	1	1	1	3	1	2	1	2	4	1	1
4a. Where do you get most of your information about AIDS?[2]											
Television................................	84	85	82	85	85	83	83	87	90	87	77
Newspapers	55	42	58	63	58	53	58	44	42	53	65
Magazines	28	26	31	24	24	31	29	20	13	26	37
Radio	10	9	12	9	12	9	10	10	11	10	9
Relatives and friends....................	9	12	10	6	9	9	8	11	9	9	9
Brochures/fliers/pamphlets	9	10	10	6	7	10	8	17	5	7	12
Doctor/HMO/clinic.......................	6	7	9	3	5	7	6	10	3	6	9
Other....................................	16	21	19	8	14	18	16	17	6	13	24
Don't know..............................	0	0	0	1	0	1	0	0	1	0	0
4b. Of the sources you just told me, from which one do you get the most information?											
Television................................	59	63	55	62	59	59	58	67	76	64	45
Newspapers	18	11	17	23	20	15	19	11	11	16	23
Magazines	8	8	9	6	6	9	8	5	3	7	12
Brochures/fliers/pamphlets	2	2	2	1	2	2	2	4	1	2	3
Doctor/HMO/clinic.......................	3	4	4	1	2	3	3	4	2	3	4
Other....................................	10	12	12	5	10	10	10	8	5	8	13
Don't know..............................	1	0	1	1	1	1	1	1	2	1	1

See footnotes at end of table.

Provisional estimates of the percent of persons 18 years of age and over with selected AIDS knowledge and attitudes from the 1987 National Health Interview Survey, by selected characteristics: United States, December 1987

[Data are based on household interviews of the civilian noninstitutionalized population. The survey design, general qualifications, and information on the reliability of the estimates are given in technical notes]

AIDS knowledge or attitude	Total	Age			Sex		Race		Education		
		18-29 years	30-49 years	50 years and over	Male	Female	White	Black	Less than 12 years	12 years	More than 12 years
5a. If you wanted more specific information about AIDS, where would you get it?[2]					Percent distribution[1]						
Doctor/HMO/clinic	60	63	59	58	59	60	59	67	58	63	58
Public health department	18	16	21	17	19	18	18	21	16	18	20
Library	12	14	13	7	11	12	12	8	5	12	14
AIDS hot line	9	12	10	5	8	9	9	12	5	9	10
Other	27	32	28	20	26	27	26	25	20	23	33
Don't know	11	7	8	17	11	10	11	10	20	10	5
5b. Which one source would you most likely use?											
Doctor/HMO/clinic	48	48	47	50	48	49	49	51	51	51	45
Public health department	13	11	15	12	13	12	13	15	11	12	14
Library	7	9	8	4	7	7	7	7	11	12	14
AIDS hot line	6	8	8	4	6	7	7	4	3	7	9
Other	14	16	15	12	14	14	14	12	4	6	7
Don't know	11	7	8	17	12	10	11	10	20	11	19
6a. A person can be infected with the AIDS virus and not have the disease AIDS.											
Definitely true	55	58	62	45	55	55	58	43	36	54	68
Probably true	24	22	23	27	24	24	24	24	26	27	20
Probably false	3	5	3	4	4	3	3	5	4	3	4
Definitely false	4	7	3	3	5	3	4	6	5	5	2
Don't know	13	9	9	22	13	14	12	21	29	12	6
6b. You can tell if people have the AIDS virus just by looking at them.											
Definitely true	1	1	1	1	1	2	1	3	2	1	1
Probably true	4	4	3	4	3	4	3	5	5	4	3
Probably false	16	17	14	18	16	17	16	16	18	17	14
Definitely false	70	74	75	62	71	70	72	63	57	70	78
Don't know	8	4	6	15	8	8	8	14	18	7	4
6c. Any person with the AIDS virus can pass it on to someone else during sexual intercourse.											
Definitely true	82	85	83	78	79	84	82	82	78	83	82
Probably true	14	12	14	16	16	12	14	12	15	14	14
Probably false	1	0	1	1	1	1	1	1	0	1	1
Definitely false	1	1	0	0	1	0	1	1	1	1	1
Don't know	3	1	2	5	3	3	3	4	7	2	2
6d. A pregnant woman who has the AIDS virus can give AIDS to her baby.											
Definitely true	77	79	79	74	74	80	77	78	73	77	79
Probably true	17	17	17	18	19	16	18	15	17	17	18
Probably false	0	0	0	0	0	0	0	0	0	0	0
Definitely false	0	0	0	0	0	0	0	1	0	0	0
Don't know	5	3	4	8	6	4	5	6	10	5	2
6e. There is a vaccine available to the public that protects a person from getting the AIDS virus.											
Definitely true	1	2	1	1	1	1	1	3	2	1	1
Probably true	3	3	2	3	3	3	2	7	5	3	2
Probably false	10	9	10	12	10	10	10	12	12	12	8
Definitely false	72	74	77	64	74	70	75	55	53	71	83
Don't know	14	11	10	21	12	16	12	23	28	14	6
6f. There is no cure for AIDS at present.											
Definitely true	86	86	88	83	86	86	87	82	77	86	90
Probably true	8	7	7	9	8	8	8	7	10	8	6
Probably false	1	1	1	1	1	1	1	1	1	1	1
Definitely false	2	3	1	1	2	1	1	2	2	2	1
Don't know	4	3	3	6	4	4	3	7	9	3	2
7. How likely do you think it is that a person will get the AIDS virus from—											
7a. Receiving a blood transfusion?											
Very likely	33	32	30	37	30	35	31	44	42	35	24
Somewhat likely	30	30	31	30	29	31	31	33	29	32	29
Somewhat unlikely	12	13	14	10	13	12	13	6	6	11	17
Very unlikely	19	20	21	15	22	16	20	7	9	16	27
Definitely not possible	2	2	1	2	1	2	2	1	2	1	2
Don't know	4	3	3	7	4	4	3	9	11	3	1
7b. Donating or giving blood?											
Very likely	8	9	7	9	9	8	7	17	15	8	5
Somewhat likely	14	15	14	14	13	14	13	22	19	14	10
Somewhat unlikely	12	14	11	11	12	11	12	12	11	13	12
Very unlikely	33	33	37	29	35	32	35	24	23	34	38
Definitely not possible	27	25	29	27	25	29	29	13	18	26	33
Don't know	6	4	4	10	6	6	5	12	15	5	2

See footnotes at end of table.

Provisional estimates of the percent of persons 18 years of age and over with selected AIDS knowledge and attitudes from the 1987 National Health Interview Survey, by selected characteristics: United States, December 1987—Con.

[Data are based on household interviews of the civilian noninstitutionalized population. The survey design, general qualifications, and information on the reliability of the estimates are given in technical notes]

AIDS knowledge or attitude	Total	Age			Sex		Race		Education		
		18-29 years	30-49 years	50 years and over	Male	Female	White	Black	Less than 12 years	12 years	More than 12 years
				Percent distribution[1]							
7c. Living near a hospital or home for AIDS patients?											
Very likely	1	1	1	1	1	1	1	2	2	1	1
Somewhat likely	4	5	3	4	4	3	3	7	5	4	2
Somewhat unlikely	8	8	8	9	9	8	7	12	9	8	8
Very unlikely	36	37	38	33	38	34	37	35	31	37	37
Definitely not possible	45	46	46	43	42	47	47	32	35	45	50
Don't know	6	4	4	11	6	6	5	11	17	5	2
7d. Working near someone with AIDS?											
Very likely	3	2	3	3	3	3	2	5	4	3	2
Somewhat likely	13	13	12	14	13	13	13	15	15	15	11
Somewhat unlikely	12	12	14	11	13	12	12	13	10	12	14
Very unlikely	34	34	36	31	35	33	35	29	27	33	39
Definitely not possible	31	34	30	29	29	32	31	28	27	32	31
Don't know	7	3	5	12	7	7	6	10	16	6	3
7e. Eating in a restaurant where the cook has AIDS?											
Very likely	8	8	7	10	8	8	7	13	12	9	5
Somewhat likely	22	24	21	23	24	20	21	25	24	24	20
Somewhat unlikely	14	16	16	11	14	14	15	12	10	14	17
Very unlikely	27	26	31	23	26	27	28	19	19	24	34
Definitely not possible	16	18	16	14	15	17	17	14	13	17	17
Don't know	12	9	9	20	12	13	12	17	23	12	6
7f. Kissing—with exchange of saliva—a person who has AIDS?											
Very likely	28	25	27	32	27	29	27	39	34	30	22
Somewhat likely	35	35	35	34	35	34	35	30	29	35	38
Somewhat unlikely	11	13	13	7	11	11	12	8	6	11	14
Very unlikely	11	13	12	8	11	11	12	7	9	9	14
Definitely not possible	5	6	5	4	5	5	5	5	5	6	4
Don't know	10	8	8	15	10	11	10	11	18	10	7
7g. Shaking hands with or touching someone who has AIDS?											
Very likely	1	1	1	2	1	2	1	3	4	1	1
Somewhat likely	7	7	6	8	8	6	6	10	10	7	5
Somewhat unlikely	14	15	15	13	16	13	14	14	12	15	14
Very unlikely	38	37	42	35	38	38	39	36	32	37	42
Definitely not possible	34	37	33	32	32	36	35	30	28	35	36
Don't know	6	3	4	11	5	6	5	8	14	5	2
7h. Sharing plates, forks, or glasses with someone who has AIDS?											
Very likely	11	10	11	11	10	11	10	17	14	12	7
Somewhat likely	28	28	27	29	29	27	27	31	29	28	26
Somewhat unlikely	14	15	14	13	15	13	14	11	10	13	17
Very unlikely	23	24	26	19	23	23	24	16	17	22	29
Definitely not possible	15	17	14	14	14	16	15	14	13	15	16
Don't know	10	6	8	14	9	10	9	11	17	10	6
7i. Using public toilets?											
Very likely	6	4	6	8	6	7	5	12	12	7	6
Somewhat likely	19	21	15	20	19	18	17	25	23	20	21
Somewhat unlikely	14	15	15	11	14	13	14	12	10	14	13
Very unlikely	30	28	34	26	30	29	31	20	18	27	29
Definitely not possible	22	25	23	19	22	22	23	18	17	21	21
Don't know	10	8	7	16	9	11	10	13	20	10	10
7j. Sharing needles for drug use with someone who has AIDS?											
Very likely	93	95	94	91	93	93	94	90	88	94	94
Somewhat likely	5	4	4	6	5	5	5	6	7	5	4
Somewhat unlikely	0	0	0	0	0	0	0	–	0	0	0
Very unlikely	0	0	0	0	0	0	0	0	0	0	0
Definitely not possible	0	0	0	–	0	0	0	0	0	0	–
Don't know	1	1	1	3	1	2	1	3	5	1	1
7k. Kissing on the cheek a person who has AIDS?											
Very likely	3	2	2	3	3	2	2	4	6	2	4
Somewhat likely	10	10	9	11	11	9	9	16	13	12	7
Somewhat unlikely	16	17	16	14	16	15	15	15	13	15	16
Very unlikely	35	35	37	34	35	36	37	28	29	35	34
Definitely not possible	30	33	31	26	27	32	30	25	24	29	33
Don't know	7	3	5	11	7	7	6	11	15	6	6
7l. Being coughed or sneezed on by someone who has AIDS?											
Very likely	8	5	8	12	8	9	8	13	14	9	7
Somewhat likely	24	26	22	25	24	24	23	28	25	26	24
Somewhat unlikely	16	17	19	13	17	16	17	15	12	16	15
Very unlikely	26	28	28	21	27	25	27	17	17	23	24
Definitely not possible	15	17	15	12	14	15	15	13	12	16	17
Don't know	11	8	8	16	11	11	10	14	21	10	12

See footnotes at end of table.

[Data are based on household interviews of the civilian noninstitutionalized population. The survey design, general qualifications, and information on the reliability of the estimates are given in technical notes]

AIDS knowledge or attitude	Total	18-29 years	30-49 years	50 years and over	Male	Female	White	Black	Less than 12 years	12 years	More than 12 years
		Age			Sex		Race		Education		
7m. Attending school with a child who has AIDS?					Percent distribution[1]						
Very likely	2	1	2	3	2	2	2	3	3	2	3
Somewhat likely	8	8	8	9	8	8	7	11	11	9	9
Somewhat unlikely	13	14	15	11	14	13	13	15	12	14	11
Very unlikely	37	36	41	33	38	36	38	30	28	35	35
Definitely not possible	31	37	29	30	30	33	32	28	26	33	34
Don't know	8	4	6	14	8	9	7	13	20	7	8
7n. Mosquitoes or other insects?											
Very likely	8	9	8	9	10	7	8	12	13	9	9
Somewhat likely	24	26	23	23	25	23	24	25	25	28	23
Somewhat unlikely	10	12	12	8	11	10	10	11	7	10	10
Very unlikely	20	21	24	16	22	19	22	14	13	18	16
Definitely not possible	16	17	16	16	16	17	17	13	13	16	18
Don't know	20	15	18	27	18	23	19	26	29	19	24
7o. Pets or animals?											
Very likely	2	1	2	2	2	2	1	5	4	2	2
Somewhat likely	9	10	7	9	10	8	8	13	12	10	8
Somewhat unlikely	10	12	9	8	10	9	10	10	7	10	8
Very unlikely	28	29	31	24	31	26	29	21	21	27	26
Definitely not possible	29	28	32	27	26	32	31	21	24	29	29
Don't know	22	19	19	30	20	24	21	31	32	22	27
7p. Having sex with a person who has AIDS?											
Very likely	94	95	95	92	93	95	94	93	91	95	96
Somewhat likely	4	4	4	5	6	3	4	4	4	4	3
Somewhat unlikely	0	0	0	0	0	0	0	0	–	0	0
Very unlikely	0	0	0	0	0	0	0	0	0	0	0
Definitely not possible	0	0	0	–	0	0	0	0	0	0	–
Don't know	1	0	1	3	1	1	1	3	4	1	1
8. Have you ever heard of a blood test for infection with the AIDS virus?											
Yes	73	78	81	59	73	73	75	58	49	74	75
No	24	20	17	36	24	24	22	38	47	23	20
Don't know	3	2	2	5	3	3	3	4	5	3	5
9. Does this test tell whether a person has the disease AIDS?											
Yes	40	43	43	34	38	41	40	37	32	43	43
No	23	26	29	15	25	22	25	12	7	20	21
Don't know	10	9	9	10	9	10	10	9	9	11	11
Never heard of test (no/don't know to q. 8)	27	22	19	41	27	27	25	42	51	26	25
10. If a person has a positive blood test for infection with the AIDS virus, does this mean that they can give someone else the AIDS virus through sexual intercourse?											
Yes	63	70	71	49	63	63	65	49	41	63	65
No	3	3	5	2	4	3	3	3	2	3	3
Don't know	6	5	6	7	6	6	6	5	6	7	7
Never heard of test (no/don't know to q. 8)	27	22	19	41	27	27	25	42	51	26	25
11. Have you ever had your blood tested for infection with the AIDS virus?											
Yes	5	7	6	2	6	4	5	9	3	5	6
Yes, in blood donation/transfusion	3	3	4	1	3	3	3	1	1	2	3
No	63	67	70	53	62	64	66	46	43	65	64
Don't know	2	1	2	2	2	1	2	1	2	1	2
Never heard of test (no/don't know to q. 8)	27	22	19	41	27	27	25	42	51	26	25
12a. Have you ever thought about having this blood test?											
Already had test	8	11	10	3	9	7	8	11	4	8	9
Yes	10	14	12	4	10	10	10	13	7	10	13
No	55	53	59	51	53	56	58	34	38	56	53
Don't know	–	–	–	–	–	–	–	–	–	–	–
Never heard of test (no/don't know to q. 8)	28	22	19	42	27	28	25	43	52	26	25
12b. Do you plan to be tested in the next 12 months?											
Already had test	8	11	10	3	9	7	8	11	4	8	9
Yes	3	6	4	1	4	3	3	8	4	3	5
No	5	5	6	2	5	5	5	2	2	4	5
Don't know	2	3	2	1	2	2	2	2	1	2	3
Never heard of test or thought about having test (no/don't know to q. 8 or q. 12a)	82	75	78	93	81	84	83	77	90	82	78

See footnotes at end of table.

Provisional estimates of the percent of persons 18 years of age and over with selected AIDS knowledge and attitudes from the 1987 National Health Interview Survey, by selected characteristics: United States, December 1987—Con.

[Data are based on household interviews of the civilian noninstitutionalized population. The survey design, general qualifications, and information on the reliability of the estimates are given in technical notes]

AIDS knowledge or attitude	Total	Age			Sex		Race		Education		
		18-29 years	30-49 years	50 years and over	Male	Female	White	Black	Less than 12 years	12 years	More than 12 years
13. Where would you go to have a blood test for the AIDS virus infection?[3]				Percent distribution[1]							
Nowhere/wouldn't take test	0	1	–	–	–	0	0	–	–	–	–
AIDS clinic	3	3	4	2	4	2	4	–	3	3	8
Other clinic	31	36	25	33	32	29	29	35	38	29	34
Doctor/HMO	45	36	50	50	40	49	46	42	30	51	41
Red Cross/blood bank	2	3	2	–	2	2	2	1	–	3	–
Other	12	11	14	7	11	13	11	16	20	6	13
Don't know	7	10	4	9	10	5	7	6	9	7	5
14. Where would you go to find out where to have this blood test?[2,4]											
AIDS hot line	11	5	31	–	10	14	14	–	13	7	20
AIDS clinic	3	–	10	–	–	7	3	–	–	–	–
Other clinic	4	–	–	21	4	3	2	17	19	–	10
Doctor/HMO	27	34	29	–	32	19	29	22	19	34	099
Friends	2	3	–	–	2	–	2	–	–	–	–
Public health department	15	8	21	32	20	7	17	10	–	18	11
Other	13	16	5	15	6	25	6	29	–	14	20
Nowhere/wouldn't take test	–	–	–	–	–	–	–	–	–	–	–
Don't know	26	34	5	32	26	25	26	22	49	27	40
15. Have you donated blood since 1985?											
Yes	13	19	16	5	16	10	13	10	5	12	18
No	87	81	84	95	84	90	87	90	95	88	82
Don't know	0	–	0	–	0	0	0	–	–	0	0
16. Have you ever personally known anyone who had the blood test for the AIDS virus infection?											
Yes	15	19	18	8	14	16	15	11	5	13	15
No	84	80	81	90	85	83	83	88	93	85	84
Don't know	2	1	2	2	2	2	2	2	2	1	2
17. What are the chances of someone you know getting the AIDS virus?											
High	9	11	12	4	8	10	9	12	6	9	9
Medium	16	21	17	11	18	14	16	16	14	16	18
Low	36	40	39	30	38	35	39	21	23	36	33
None	26	19	22	36	23	29	25	29	34	27	27
Refused	0	0	0	0	0	0	0	0	0	0	0
Don't know	13	8	10	19	13	12	11	22	23	12	13
18. What are your chances of getting the AIDS virus?											
High	1	1	1	0	1	1	1	2	1	1	1
Medium	3	4	4	3	4	3	3	4	4	3	4
Low	29	36	33	20	31	28	30	21	18	26	30
None	62	55	59	72	60	63	62	65	69	65	59
Refused	0	0	0	0	0	0	0	–	0	0	0
Don't know	4	4	3	5	4	4	3	8	9	4	7
19. Here are methods some people use to prevent getting the AIDS virus through sexual activity. How effective is—											
19a. Using a diaphragm?											
Very effective	2	3	2	2	3	2	2	5	3	2	2
Somewhat effective	11	12	10	12	11	12	11	13	11	12	9
Not at all effective	57	58	67	46	56	58	60	44	37	57	59
Don't know how effective	23	20	17	32	24	22	22	26	35	23	20
Don't know method	6	7	4	9	7	6	5	12	15	5	11
19b. Using a condom?											
Very effective	36	41	37	30	37	34	37	32	28	35	34
Somewhat effective	47	47	50	45	47	47	48	41	39	48	47
Not at all effective	6	5	6	7	5	7	5	10	8	6	6
Don't know how effective	10	7	6	16	9	10	9	14	19	9	9
Don't know method	2	1	1	4	1	2	2	4	6	1	4
19c. Using a spermicidal jelly, foam, or cream?											
Very effective	2	3	2	1	2	1	1	3	2	2	4
Somewhat effective	14	15	15	11	14	14	14	13	8	14	11
Not at all effective	56	58	63	47	55	57	58	46	43	55	57
Don't know how effective	22	18	17	32	23	22	22	27	34	23	20
Don't know method	6	6	4	9	6	6	5	11	12	5	8
19d. Being celibate, that is, not having sex at all?											
Very effective	91	91	94	88	91	91	92	89	84	92	89
Somewhat effective	4	5	3	5	4	4	4	5	5	4	4
Not at all effective	1	2	1	1	1	1	1	1	1	1	1
Don't know how effective	3	2	2	4	3	3	3	3	7	2	3
Don't know method	1	1	0	1	0	1	1	1	3	1	2

See footnotes at end of table.

Provisional estimates of the percent of persons 18 years of age and over with selected AIDS knowledge and attitudes from the 1987 National Health Interview Survey, by selected characteristics: United States, December 1987—Con.

[Data are based on household interviews of the civilian noninstitutionalized population. The survey design, general qualifications, and information on the reliability of the estimates are given in technical notes]

AIDS knowledge or attitude	Total	Age			Sex		Race		Education		
		18-29 years	30-49 years	50 years and over	Male	Female	White	Black	Less than 12 years	12 years	More than 12 years
19e. Two people who do not have the AIDS virus having a completely monogamous relationship, that is, having sex only with each other?					Percent distribution[1]						
Very effective	86	86	91	82	87	85	88	78	76	88	82
Somewhat effective	8	8	6	9	7	8	7	11	9	7	8
Not at all effective	1	2	1	1	2	1	1	3	2	2	2
Don't know how effective	4	3	2	7	3	4	3	6	9	3	6
Don't know method	1	1	1	2	1	2	1	2	4	1	1
20. Have you ever discussed AIDS with a friend or relative?											
Yes	65	71	74	49	61	69	65	68	44	63	65
No	35	28	25	50	39	31	34	32	56	36	34
Don't know	0	0	0	1	0	1	0	0	1	0	1
21. When was the last time you discussed AIDS with a friend or relative?											
0-3 days ago	14	14	16	11	13	15	13	18	10	14	16
4-7 days ago	15	17	18	11	15	16	15	18	10	15	16
8-14 days ago	8	9	10	5	8	8	8	5	6	8	8
15-31 days ago	14	17	15	10	13	15	14	13	9	14	10
More than 31 days ago	9	11	10	6	8	10	9	9	5	8	11
Never discussed (no/don't know to q. 20)	36	29	27	52	40	32	36	33	58	37	36
Don't know	4	4	4	5	4	4	4	4	4	4	3
24. Have you ever discussed AIDS with [any of your children age 10-17]?[5]											
Yes	62	59	63	56	50	73	64	57	49	61	66
No	38	41	37	44	50	27	36	43	51	39	34
Don't know	–	–	–	–	–	–	–	–	–	–	–
25. Have your children had any instruction at school about AIDS?[5]											
Yes	51	38	50	66	49	52	49	63	47	50	52
No	19	44	20	10	18	21	21	13	20	20	19
Don't know	30	17	31	25	33	27	31	24	32	29	29
26. Have you ever personally known anyone with the AIDS virus?											
Yes	7	7	10	5	6	8	7	9	4	5	7
No	91	92	88	94	92	90	91	87	95	93	92
Don't know	2	2	2	2	2	2	1	4	2	1	1
27. Have you ever personally known anyone with AIDS?											
Yes	7	6	10	5	6	8	7	10	4	5	6
No	91	93	89	94	92	91	92	88	94	93	93
Don't know	1	1	1	1	2	1	1	2	1	1	1
28. The U.S. Public Health Service has said that AIDS is one of the major health problems in the country but exactly how many people it affects is not known. The Surgeon General has proposed that a study be conducted and blood samples be taken to help find out how widespread the problem is. If you were selected in this national sample of people to have their blood tested with assurances of privacy of test results, would you have the test?											
Yes	70	75	73	63	71	69	71	70	64	70	70
No	21	19	18	26	21	21	21	19	24	22	21
Other	2	2	2	2	2	2	2	2	2	2	2
Don't know	7	4	7	8	6	8	6	9	9	6	8
29. Would you want to know the results of the blood test?[6]											
Yes	98	98	98	97	98	98	98	98	98	99	97
No	2	1	1	2	2	2	2	1	2	1	2
Don't know	1	1	1	0	0	1	0	1	1	1	1

[1] Excludes persons for whom no response was recorded or who refused to respond. For question 2 through 27, total also excludes persons who never heard of AIDS.
[2] Muliple responses may sum to more than 100 percent.
[3] Based on persons answering yes to question 12a.
[4] Based on persons answering don't know to question 13.
[5] Based on persons answering yes to question 22, Do you have any children aged 10-17? Question 23 was, How many do you have?
[6] Based on persons answering yes to question 28.

NOTE: Total, age, sex, and education include persons of other and unknown race not shown separately under race. Education refers to years of school completed.

Source: "AIDS Knowledge and Attitudes for December 1987: Provisional Data From the National Health Interview Survey," nchs advancedata, National Center for Health Statistics, May 16, 1988)

Two out of three adults had discussed AIDS with friends or relatives. Those over 50 years of age were least likely to have discussed it. Sixty percent of parents with children between the ages of 10 and 17 had talked with their children about AIDS. Of those with children in that age range, 51 percent reported that their children received instruction about AIDS at school.

Nationwide Test

When asked about the prospect of a national sample of testing, with assurances of privacy, to determine how widespread the problem is, 7 out of 10 responded that they would have the test. Of those who responded yes, 98 percent said they would want to know the results.

RACIAL DIFFERENCES IN POLLS

As indicated above, the National Health Interview Survey illustrated the differences among minorities in term of knowledge of the disease, methods of transmission, and testing procedures. In addition, Dr. Susan Blake of the American Red Cross National Headquarters has examined all published opinion polls on AIDS since 1983 to analyze the differences in responses between the races.

Her preliminary analysis found that, based on a 1987 Gallup Poll of 1,015 New Yorkers, 28 percent of the white respondents believed you could get AIDS from donating blood, while 54 percent of blacks and 60 percent of Hispanics shared the same view. All, however, were aware of the risks of sharing needles and sexual activity among homosexual men.

Because many minorities believe that casual contact can transmit the AIDS virus, it is not surprising that many minority individuals feel more personally vulnerable than whites. Thirty-two percent of those minorities polled in 1987 felt personally vulnerable, fearful, and concerned about AIDS, compared with 15 percent of whites. Subsequent polls by the Illinois Department of Public Health and the Los Angeles Times also found AIDS anxiety higher among blacks.

Interestingly, minorities reported a higher level of interest in reading or watching programs about AIDS. Forty-two percent of whites interviewed by various polls said they would read an entire article or watch an entire program about AIDS, while 64 percent of minorities said they would. When asked about changes in sexual behavior as a result of the AIDS threat, 4 percent of whites reported changing their behavior in an effort to protect themselves, while 25 percent of minorities indicated that they had also. These changes seem to refer to limiting sexual partners.

WE'RE SORRY, BUT...

A series of questions put to the American public by The Gallup Poll July 10-13, 1987 brought responses that revealed a high degree of compassion for persons with AIDS. More than three-quarters (78 percent) of those who responded to the telephone interview felt that AIDS victims should be treated with compassion. Almost half (48 percent) believed those with AIDS should be allowed to live normal lives in the community. Only one-third thought employers should have the right to dismiss someone with AIDS because of their disease.

However, those questioned disagreed strongly over whether AIDS is a punishment for declining moral standards. Forty-two percent of those polled agreed, while an almost equal proportion (43 percent) disagreed. Somewhat less than half (45 percent) thought that most of those with AIDS had only themselves to blame. This undoubtedly reflects a negative attitude towards those who participate in homosexual/bisexual activities, casual sex, and drug use lifestyles, since these persons are more likely than others to be infected. However, 41 percent refused to agree or disagree that AIDS victims were to blame for their illness. There was considerable agreement, however, on the subject of card-carrying to identify an AIDS victims. Sixty percent thought that people with AIDS should be required to carry a card to that effect. A method of identifying those who are infected is considered a very real problem for sexually active singles who are not in monogamous (with only one other person) relationships.

The most obvious differences of opinion were between those who were Evangelical Christians and those who were not, and among respondents from contrasting educational backgrounds. Evangelicals were more likely to feel persons with AIDS were to blame for their condition and to view AIDS as a moral indictment.

Similarly, those who were non-high school graduates were more likely to hold "only themselves to blame" and punishment for moral decline views than those who were college graduates. Colleges graduates were also far more likely than those without a college background to favor permitting AIDS sufferers a normal life in the community.

A similar poll conducted for The Bradman Charitable Foundation by Social Surveys (Gallup Poll) Limited found that the British and American public held many similar attitudes on AIDS. The British, however, were more tolerant of AIDS victims remaining in the community, and were more likely to support the carrying of mandatory cards.

Premarital Sex and Disease

Between 1969 and 1985, the percentage of those interviewed by the Gallup

Beliefs about AIDS Victims
(Based on views of Americans)

	Agree	Disagree	Neither agree nor disagree	No opinion
AIDS suffers should be treated with compassion	78%	7%	13%	2%
People with AIDS should be allowed to live in the community normally	48	29	19	4
Employers should have the right to dismiss an employee because that person has AIDS	33	43	19	5
Most people with AIDS have only themselves to blame	45	13	41	1
I sometimes think that AIDS is a punishment for the decline in moral standards	42	43	12	3
People with the AIDS virus should be made to carry a card to this effect	60	24	13	3

Beliefs about AIDS Victims
(Percent agreeing)

	Americans	British
AIDS sufferers should be treated with compassion	78%	75%
People with AIDS should be allowed to live in the community normally	48	61
People with the AIDS virus should be made to carry a card to this effect	60	71
I sometimes think that AIDS is a punishment for the decline in moral standards	42	35
Most people with AIDS have only themselves to blame	45	46
Employers should have the right to dismiss an employee because that person has AIDS	33	28

Source: The Gallup Poll, Princeton, NJ

121

Are Victims to Blame?

QUESTION: I am going to read you a list of statements that have been made about people with AIDS. For each statement please tell me whether you agree or disagree by using one of the responses on this card. Most people with AIDS have only themselves to blame.

July 10-13, 1987 (Personal)

	Agree strongly	Agree	Neither agree nor disagree	Disagree	Disagree strongly	No opinion	Number of Interviews
NATIONAL	14%	31%	13%	29%	12%	1%	1,607
SEX							
Men	17	31	13	27	10	2	806
Women	12	31	13	30	13	2	801
AGE							
18-29 years	12	31	11	32	14	*	298
18-24 years	12	31	15	30	11	*	164
25-29 years	13	32	5	33	17	*	134
30-49 years	13	26	14	31	15	1	642
50 & older	18	36	13	24	6	3	663
50-64 years	16	35	11	28	8	2	350
65 & older	21	38	14	19	4	4	313
REGION							
East	16	30	11	30	12	1	384
Midwest	15	30	16	28	10	1	420
South	13	37	13	26	9	2	484
West	15	23	11	32	18	1	319
RACE							
Whites	14	31	13	28	12	*	1,425
Non-whites	17	28	12	31	12	2	182
Blacks	17	26	12	33	11	1	166
Hispanics	16	43	9	25	6	1	96
EDUCATION							
College graduates	12	26	15	29	18	*	370
College incomplete	12	27	14	32	15	*	403
High school graduates	14	32	12	33	8	1	514
Not high school grads.	20	38	11	19	8	4	319
POLITICS							
Republicans	17	34	12	27	8	2	488
Democrats	14	32	12	28	13	1	688
Independents	13	26	13	33	14	1	402
OCCUPATION OF CWE							
Professional & business	11	27	13	34	15	*	481
Other white collar	15	32	13	25	15	*	115
Blue collar	14	31	12	31	11	1	582
Skilled workers	14	30	14	29	12	1	300
Unskilled workers	14	32	10	32	10	2	282
HOUSEHOLD INCOME							
$40,000 & over	12	29	12	32	14	1	366
$25,000-$39,999	15	29	11	31	13	1	390
$15,000-$24,999	12	33	17	27	9	2	327
Under $15,000	19	33	11	25	11	1	438
RELIGION							
Protestants	14	35	13	27	10	1	916
Catholics	16	28	12	32	11	1	476
LABOR UNION							
Labor-union families	12	28	10	33	16	1	306
Non-union families	15	32	14	28	10	1	1,301
EVANGELICALS							
Evangelicals	17	40	12	24	6	1	435
Non-evangelicals	14	28	13	31	13	1	1,132

*Less than one percent.

Survey 278-Q. 14B

Is AIDS a Moral Punishment?

QUESTION: I am going to read you a list of statements that have been made about people with AIDS. For each statement please tell me whether you agree or disagree by using one of the responses on this card. I sometimes think that AIDS is a punishment for the decline in moral standards.

July 10-13, 1987 (Personal)

	Agree strongly	Agree	Neither agree nor disagree	Disagree	Disagree strongly	No opinion	Number of Interviews
NATIONAL	16%	26%	12%	25%	18%	3%	1,607
SEX							
Men	15	27	13	25	17	3	806
Women	17	24	12	26	18	3	801
AGE							
18-29 years	13	26	13	26	22	*	298
18-24 years	12	26	17	27	18	*	164
25-29 years	16	26	8	25	25	*	134
30-49 years	15	23	11	26	20	*	642
50 & older	20	28	11	24	12	5	663
50-64 years	22	25	10	25	15	3	350
65 & older	19	31	12	23	9	6	313
REGION							
East	13	18	12	33	23	1	384
Midwest	13	27	15	27	16	2	420
South	22	31	14	17	12	4	484
West	14	27	8	26	22	3	319
RACE							
Whites	16	25	12	25	19	3	1,425
Non-whites	20	30	11	24	12	3	182
Blacks	20	29	13	25	9	3	166
Hispanics	18	31	14	21	7	2	96
EDUCATION							
College graduates	9	23	13	26	29	2	370
College incomplete	13	22	11	29	24	4	403
High school graduates	19	27	13	25	13	3	514
Not high school grads.	23	30	12	21	7	7	319
POLITICS							
Republicans	17	28	12	25	17	1	488
Democrats	17	26	13	23	17	4	688
Independents	15	23	10	29	21	2	402
OCCUPATION OF CWE							
Professional & business	11	20	13	28	26	2	481
Other white collar	14	28	11	22	24	3	115
Blue collar	18	28	13	24	14	3	582
Skilled workers	19	30	13	22	14	2	300
Unskilled workers	16	26	13	27	14	4	282
HOUSEHOLD INCOME							
$40,000 & over	10	21	10	31	27	1	366
$25,000-$39,999	17	24	17	24	17	1	390
$15,000-$24,999	18	29	10	23	16	4	327
Under $15,000	19	28	12	26	11	4	438
RELIGION							
Protestants	19	29	13	23	13	3	916
Catholics	12	23	12	30	20	3	476
LABOR UNION							
Labor-union families	17	26	9	28	19	1	306
Non-union families	16	26	13	25	17	3	1,301
EVANGELICALS							
Evangelicals	26	34	12	17	8	3	435
Non-evangelicals	13	23	12	28	22	2	1,132

*Less than one percent.

Survey 278-Q. 14A

Source: The Gallup Poll, Princeton, NJ

Employer Tolerance of Victims

QUESTION: *I am going to read you a list of statements that have been made about people with AIDS. For each statement please tell me whether you agree or disagree by using one of the responses on this card. Employers should have the right to dismiss an employee because that person has AIDS.*

July 10-13, 1987 (Personal)

	Agree strongly	Agree	Neither agree nor disagree	Disagree	Disagree strongly	No opinion	Number of Interviews
NATIONAL	9%	24%	19%	32%	11%	5%	1,607
SEX							
Men	10	25	17	34	9	5	806
Women	7	23	23	31	12	4	801
AGE							
18-29 years	7	20	23	34	13	3	298
18-24 years	8	23	23	32	10	4	164
25-29 years	5	17	23	35	17	3	134
30-49 years	9	22	19	33	13	4	642
50 & older	9	28	18	31	7	6	663
50-64 years	9	25	22	32	7	5	350
65 & older	10	33	14	30	5	8	313
REGION							
East	10	22	16	39	10	3	384
Midwest	6	25	21	35	10	3	420
South	11	28	23	26	6	8	484
West	9	22	18	29	18	4	319
RACE							
Whites	9	24	20	31	11	5	1,425
Non-whites	6	24	16	42	9	3	182
Blacks	5	25	14	44	9	4	166
Hispanics	14	25	14	35	6	6	96
EDUCATION							
College graduates	7	20	22	30	18	3	370
College incomplete	8	23	23	32	11	3	403
High school graduates	9	26	18	34	9	4	514
Not high school grads.	12	26	15	31	7	9	319
POLITICS							
Republicans	10	26	23	29	8	4	488
Democrats	7	22	18	35	12	6	688
Independents	10	26	17	31	12	4	402
OCCUPATION OF CWE							
Professional & business	9	22	19	34	13	3	481
Other white collar	7	17	22	37	14	3	115
Blue collar	7	24	21	32	10	6	582
Skilled workers	7	29	21	30	9	4	300
Unskilled workers	8	19	21	35	10	7	282
HOUSEHOLD INCOME							
$40,000 & over	8	20	21	33	15	3	366
$25,000-$39,999	9	23	18	33	13	3	390
$15,000-$24,999	8	20	25	34	7	6	327
Under $15,000	10	31	15	31	8	5	438
RELIGION							
Protestants	9	26	20	32	8	5	916
Catholics	8	24	16	36	12	4	476
LABOR UNION							
Labor-union families	8	23	16	36	12	5	306
Non-union families	9	24	21	31	10	5	1,301
EVANGELICALS							
Evangelicals	12	30	21	25	8	4	435
Non-evangelicals	8	22	19	35	12	4	1,132

*Less than one percent.

Survey 278-G, Q. 13H

Community Tolerance of Victims

QUESTION: *I am going to read you a list of statements that have been made about people with AIDS. For each statement please tell me whether you agree or disagree by using one of the responses on this card. People with AIDS should be allowed to live in the community normally.*

July 10-13, 1987 (Personal)

	Agree strongly	Agree	Neither agree nor disagree	Disagree	Disagree strongly	No opinion	Number of Interviews
NATIONAL	8%	40%	19%	21%	8%	4%	1,607
SEX							
Men	9	38	18	22	9	4	806
Women	8	42	20	19	7	4	801
AGE							
18-29 years	12	43	19	16	9	1	298
18-24 years	11	42	17	16	12	2	164
25-29 years	13	44	21	17	4	1	134
30-49 years	8	38	20	23	8	3	642
50 & older	6	40	19	20	7	8	663
50-64 years	5	43	17	20	9	6	350
65 & older	6	36	21	21	5	11	313
REGION							
East	10	41	18	19	7	5	384
Midwest	7	47	20	17	6	3	420
South	6	31	20	26	11	6	484
West	12	44	18	17	7	2	319
RACE							
Whites	8	40	19	20	8	5	1,425
Non-whites	10	37	18	24	8	3	182
Blacks	9	38	16	25	8	4	166
Hispanics	10	38	14	24	11	3	96
EDUCATION							
College graduates	13	50	18	14	3	2	370
College incomplete	7	42	20	21	8	2	403
High school graduates	8	36	21	21	9	5	514
Not high school grads.	7	34	16	24	10	9	319
POLITICS							
Republicans	6	37	20	25	8	4	488
Democrats	10	41	16	20	7	6	688
Independents	8	41	23	17	8	3	402
OCCUPATION OF CWE							
Professional & business	9	47	16	19	6	3	481
Other white collar	11	41	24	19	4	1	115
Blue collar	6	39	20	21	8	6	582
Skilled workers	6	38	21	23	8	4	300
Unskilled workers	9	40	20	18	8	5	282
HOUSEHOLD INCOME							
$40,000 & over	11	45	20	15	6	3	366
$25,000-$39,999	7	41	21	19	9	3	390
$15,000-$24,999	7	40	18	24	7	4	327
Under $15,000	8	37	18	22	9	6	438
RELIGION							
Protestants	7	38	20	22	8	5	916
Catholics	8	45	17	19	7	4	476
LABOR UNION							
Labor-union families	7	41	21	18	7	6	306
Non-union families	8	40	19	21	8	4	1,301
EVANGELICALS							
Evangelicals	6	34	21	22	11	6	435
Non-evangelicals	9	42	19	20	7	3	1,132

*Less than one percent.

Survey 278-G, Q. 14C

Source: The Gallup Poll, Princeton, NJ

sexual attitudes are changing in this country. What is your opinion about this: Do you think it is wrong for a man and a woman to have sexual relations before marriage, or not?

| | July 10-13, 1987 (Personal) | | | |
	Wrong	Not wrong	No opinion	Number of Interviews
NATIONAL	46%	48%	6%	1,607
SEX				
Men	39	55	6	806
Women	53	41	6	801
AGE				
18-24 years	27	70	3	298
25-29 years	27	69	4	164
30-49 years	41	57	2	642
50 & older	65	27	8	663
50-64 years	59	33	8	350
65 & older	70	21	9	313
REGION				
East	37	58	5	384
Midwest	42	52	6	420
South	61	32	7	484
West	40	56	4	319
RACE				
Whites	46	48	6	1,425
Non-whites	47	47	6	182
Blacks	48	45	7	166
Hispanics	47	50	3	96
EDUCATION				
College graduates	37	60	3	370
College incomplete	42	53	5	403
High school graduates	45	47	8	514
Not high school grads.	60	34	6	319
POLITICS				
Republicans	50	46	4	488
Democrats	47	47	6	688
Independents	41	53	6	402
OCCUPATION OF CWE				
Professional & business	37	59	4	481
Other white collar	39	54	7	115
Blue collar	45	49	6	582
Skilled workers	43	52	5	300
Unskilled workers	46	46	8	282
HOUSEHOLD INCOME				
$40,000 & over	38	56	6	366
$25,000-$39,999	41	56	3	390
$15,000-$24,999	47	45	8	327
Under $15,000	56	38	6	438
RELIGION				
Protestants	52	42	6	916
Catholics	39	56	5	476
LABOR UNION				
Labor-union families	45	51	4	306
Non-union families	46	48	6	1,301
EVANGELICALS				
Evangelicals	70	25	5	435
Non-evangelicals	37	57	6	1,132

Premarital Sex

	Wrong	Not wrong	No opinion
1987	46%	48%	6%
1985	39	52	9
1973	48	43	9
1969	68	21	11

Compassion for Victims

QUESTION: *I am going to read you a list of statements that have been made about people with AIDS. For each statement please tell me whether you agree or disagree by using one of the responses on this card. AIDS sufferers should be treated with compassion.*

| | July 10-13, 1987 (Personal) | | | | | | |
	Agree strongly	Agree	Neither agree nor disagree	Disagree	Disagree strongly	No opinion	Number of Interviews
NATIONAL	26%	52%	13%	5%	2%	2%	1,607
SEX							
Men	23	51	14	7	2	3	806
Women	28	53	12	4	2	1	801
AGE							
18-24 years	24	48	17	7	2	2	298
25-29 years	18	53	16	8	4	*	164
30-49 years	32	42	13	7	4	2	642
50 & older	30	49	11	6	2	2	663
50-64 years	23	50	17	6	3	1	350
65 & older	20	57	10	8	1	4	313
REGION							
East	30	51	10	6	2	1	384
Midwest	22	54	13	6	3	2	420
South	20	50	17	6	3	4	484
West	32	54	10	1	2	1	319
RACE							
Whites	25	52	14	5	2	2	1,425
Non-whites	29	50	10	7	3	1	182
Blacks	26	52	10	6	3	3	166
Hispanics	24	47	17	7	1	4	96
EDUCATION							
College graduates	38	53	7	1	1	*	370
College incomplete	28	52	12	6	1	1	403
High school graduates	21	51	17	6	2	3	514
Not high school grads.	18	53	17	7	3	2	319
POLITICS							
Republicans	21	54	14	5	4	2	488
Democrats	26	52	13	5	2	2	688
Independents	31	51	10	4	2	2	402
OCCUPATION OF CWE							
Professional & business	30	55	10	2	2	1	481
Other white collar	32	44	13	7	2	2	115
Blue collar	24	50	15	6	2	3	582
Skilled workers	27	50	16	4	2	1	300
Unskilled workers	22	50	14	8	3	3	282
HOUSEHOLD INCOME							
$40,000 & over	31	55	10	2	2	*	366
$25,000-$39,999	26	52	14	5	2	1	390
$15,000-$24,999	21	51	18	6	1	3	327
Under $15,000	24	50	12	8	3	3	438
RELIGION							
Protestants	23	55	13	5	2	2	916
Catholics	26	52	12	6	2	2	476
LABOR UNION							
Labor-union families	27	52	12	4	3	2	306
Non-union families	25	52	13	6	2	2	1,301
EVANGELICALS							
Evangelicals	21	56	11	5	4	3	435
Non-evangelicals	27	51	14	5	2	1	1,132

*Less than one percent.

Survey #276-G, Q. 14E

Source: The Gallup Poll, Princeton, NJ

Casual Transmission of AIDS
(Based on those aware of AIDS)

QUESTION: Do you believe a person can get AIDS by being in a crowded place with someone who has it?

	Yes, can	No, cannot	Not sure	Number of Interviews
		March 7-10, 1986		
NATIONAL	6%	81%	13%	990
SEX				
Men	7	79	14	492
Women	4	83	13	498
AGE				
18-29 years	8	86	6	258
30-49 years	5	86	9	427
Total 50 & older	5	73	22	298
50-64 years	5	78	17	177
65 & older	6	65	29	121
REGION				
East	3	86	11	255
Midwest	6	81	13	250
South	6	77	17	301
West	6	83	11	184
RACE				
Whites	5	82	13	880
Non-whites	10	79	11	110
Blacks	11	76	13	76
EDUCATION				
College graduates	2	91	7	290
College incomplete	5	87	8	238
High school graduates	5	82	13	346
Not high school grads.	11	62	27	112
POLITICS				
Republicans	5	81	14	330
Democrats	6	80	14	270
Independents	6	83	11	346
HOUSEHOLD INCOME				
$35,000 & over	7	87	6	242
$15,000-$34,999	4	85	11	448
Under $15,000	8	72	20	230
RELIGION				
Protestants	6	80	14	596
Catholics	4	85	11	234

Permit Child to Attend School With AIDS Victim?
(Based on those aware of AIDS)

QUESTION: A 14-year-old Indiana boy who contracted AIDS through a contaminated blood transfusion was banned from attending school classes. After a county medical officer ruled that he posed no health threat to his classmates, he went back to school, but the parents of almost half the students at his school kept their children home. If you had children of this age, would you permit them to attend classes with a child who had AIDS, or not?

	Would permit them to attend	Would not permit attendance	No opinion	Number of Interviews
		March 7-10, 1986		
NATIONAL	67%	24%	9%	990
SEX				
Men	66	27	7	492
Women	67	22	11	498
AGE				
18-29 years	65	29	6	258
30-49 years	69	23	8	427
Total 50 & older	65	23	12	298
50-64 years	71	20	9	177
65 & older	57	27	16	121
REGION				
East	64	27	9	255
Midwest	69	20	11	250
South	63	27	10	301
West	72	22	6	184
RACE				
Whites	67	24	9	880
Non-whites	64	27	9	110
Blacks	60	31	9	76
EDUCATION				
College graduates	72	19	9	290
College incomplete	68	23	9	238
High school graduates	67	23	10	346
Not high school grads.	57	35	8	112
POLITICS				
Republicans	67	25	8	330
Democrats	67	24	9	270
Independents	68	23	9	346
HOUSEHOLD INCOME				
$35,000 & over	64	26	10	242
$15,000-$34,999	71	23	6	448
Under $15,000	64	25	11	230
RELIGION				
Protestants	67	25	8	596
Catholics	71	21	8	234

Source: The Gallup Poll, Princeton, NJ

Poll who said premarital sex was wrong dropped 29 percentage points from 68 percent to 39 percent. However, in only the two years to 1987, it rose to 46 percent, an indication of a reversal on the liberal views towards premarital sex. Researchers speculate that, in addition to the resurgence of moral standards by many religious groups, fear of sexually-transmitted diseases, including, or perhaps, especially AIDS, may be a contributing factor. Females and older respondents were more likely than males and younger persons to believe sex before marriage was not right.

When questioned further about why sex before marriage was wrong, of those who responded that it was, interesting differences

Premarital Sex
(Percent saying "wrong")

	1987	1985	1969
NATIONAL	46%	39%	68%
Men	39	32	62
Women	53	44	74
18-29 years	27	18	49
30-49 years	41	35	67
50 & older	65	56	80
Protestants	52	46	70
Catholics	39	33	72
College education	40	31	56
High school	42	40	69
Grade school	60	60	77
East	37	40	65
Midwest	42	36	69
South	61	48	78
West	40	24	55

Why Premarital Sex Is Wrong
(Based on those who say premarital sex is wrong)
QUESTION: *Why do you feel this way?*

July 10–13, 1987 (Personal)

	Moral, religious reasons	Risk of disease	Risk of pregnancy	Women should be virgins before marriage	Other	No opinion	Number of interviews
NATIONAL	**83%**	**20%**	**13%**	**9%**	**5%**	**3%**	**762**
SEX							
Men	85	18	11	6	4	3	340
Women	82	21	14	10	6	3	422
AGE							
18-29 years	75	27	17	17	6	2	80
18-24 years	70	27	20	16	8	2	46
25-29 years	82	26	13	18	4	2	34
30-49 years	80	27	15	7	4	4	259
50 & older	88	13	9	7	5	3	422
50-64 years	87	11	5	6	8	2	206
65 & older	89	15	14	9	1	4	216
REGION							
East	71	22	14	7	5	5	140
Midwest	88	15	10	2	6	1	185
South	89	21	15	12	2	2	303
West	79	20	8	9	8	6	134
RACE							
Whites	84	21	12	8	5	3	678
Non-whites	81	13	18	15	2	4	84
Blacks	83	12	17	15	2	4	77
Hispanics	63	33	21	17	10	6	49
EDUCATION							
College graduates	89	22	11	7	6	2	143
College incomplete	81	18	17	6	8	4	180
High school graduates	84	21	9	7	3	3	245
Not high school grads.	81	19	14	13	4	3	193
POLITICS							
Republicans	85	23	13	8	6	3	255
Democrats	83	17	13	10	3	4	329
Independents	82	23	12	7	7	1	165
OCCUPATION OF CWE							
Professional & business	86	17	13	6	9	5	188
Other white collar	71	38	22	9	3	*	46
Blue collar	80	24	13	10	3	2	267
Skilled workers	82	24	12	9	6	*	132
Unskilled workers	78	23	14	10	2	3	135
HOUSEHOLD INCOME							
$40,000 & over	86	25	13	7	7	1	136
$25,000-$39,999	86	19	12	7	4	3	172
$15,000-$24,999	78	18	9	3	6	5	160
Under $15,000	34	17	14	13	4	3	254
RELIGION							
Protestants	88	18	12	8	4	3	489
Catholics	90	15	11	13	1	2	197
LABOR UNION							
Labor-union families	82	21	12	2	7	2	134
Non-union families	84	20	13	10	4	3	628
EVANGELICALS							
Evangelicals	91	19	9	10	4	2	307
Non-evangelicals	77	21	15	7	6	3	435

Source: The Gallup Poll, Princeton, NJ

between the ages emerged. Younger adults, those 18-49 years of age, were almost twice as likely as those 50 years or older to cite risk of disease. Adults in the 18-49 age group were most likely to be unmarried and have more practical reasons for being opposed to premarital sex. The overwhelming justifications for not having sex before marriage were religious and moral reasons.

AWARENESS, TRANSMISSION, AND SCHOOL CHILDREN

A March 1986 Gallup Poll found that 98 percent of those polled knew about AIDS, and that a very small proportion, 6 percent, believed AIDS could be transmitted simply by being in a public place with someone who has it. Of the overwhelming majority who were aware of AIDS, two-thirds (67 percent) would allow their children to attend school with a student who has AIDS, while one-fourth would not. Of this latter group, only 17 percent thought the disease could be casually transmitted, almost 60 percent did not believe it could be casually transmitted, and 24 percent were undecided. In spite of what they knew and felt, they were still apprehensive about the disease. Older, less well educated, and less-affluent respondents tended to be less sure of the methods of AIDS transmission, and less likely than their counterparts to allow their children to attend school with a child who has AIDS.

QUESTION: Have you heard or read about the disease called AIDS - acquired immune deficiency syndrome?

| | March 7-10, 1986 | | |
	Yes	No	Number of Interviews
NATIONAL	**98%**	**2%**	**1,004**
SEX			
Men	98	2	499
Women	98	2	505
AGE			
18-29 years	99	1	261
30-49 years	99	1	430
Total 50 & older	97	3	306
50-64 years	99	1	180
65 & older	94	6	126
REGION			
East	99	1	257
Midwest	98	2	253
South	97	3	308
West	99	1	186
RACE			
Whites	99	1	889
Non-whites	95	5	115
Blacks	96	4	78
EDUCATION			
College graduates	99	1	291
College incomplete	99	1	241
High school graduates	99	1	351
Not high school grads.	95	5	117
POLITICS			
Republicans	99	1	332
Democrats	97	3	276
Independents	99	1	351
HOUSEHOLD INCOME			
$35,000 & over	99	1	243
$15,000-$34,999	99	1	454
Under $15,000	97	3	235
RELIGION			
Protestants	98	2	602
Catholics	98	2	239

Source: The Gallup Poll, Princeton, NJ

CHAPTER XIV

THE COMMISSION REPORT

The FY88 Budget has called for the establishment of a special AIDS agency, led by an AIDS "czar" under the direction of the Office of the Assistant Secretary of Health (OASH). From that office, the Congress hoped, would come a long overdue national policy on AIDS, giving direction on control of the disease, spending for research and education, and the overall impact of the epidemic. Until such an office is established, however, many observers hope the President will follow the recommendations of the Presidential Commission on the Human Immunodeficency Virus Epidemic.

The Commission's Charge

The Commission, created by President Ronald Reagan in 1987, was fraught with controversy from its beginnings. Critics claimed that few on the panel had first-hand knowledge of AIDS and that no one with AIDS was on the commission. The first chairman resigned not long after his appointment. The appointment of Admiral James D. Watkins, USN (Ret.) seemed to have brought considerable respect to a Commission that many saw as little more than political window dressing. Admiral Watkins brought order to the Commission and treated those involved with respect. Despite the earlier problems, the Commission was able to hold more than 40 hearings and hear testimony from over 600 witnesses. On June 24, 1988, the Commission presented its final report to the President, a year after it was formed. While various groups have questioned particular findings, the overall conclusions and recommendations listed below have won general approval.

The Commission was presented with an unusual, and sometimes unpleasant, view of some of American life. They saw first-hand the horrors of drug abuse, the overburdened health care system, the inadequate search for a cure or a vaccine, the lack of proper education in our schools, and the rejection, condemnation, and discrimination of Persons With AIDS (PWA, as they prefer to be called).

IMPORTANT FINDINGS AND RECOMMENDATIONS

Following are the 20 most important findings. The recommendations, if followed could provide a comprehensive national strategy for effectively managing the HIV epidemic.

1. The term "HIV infection" more correctly defines the problem than the obsolete term "AIDS." The focus of everyone's attention should be on the

course of the HIV infection, rather than the later stages of ARC (AIDS Related Complex) and AIDS. The commission feels that concentration on the later stages has hampered the ability to deal with the epidemic, and that federal and state data collection efforts should be focused on early HIV reports.

2. In keeping with the first recommendation, the Commission calls for early diagnosis of HIV infection. Not only does this allow for proper medical treatment and counseling, but for proper follow-up by public health officials. HIV, though unique in other ways, resembles other chronic conditions in that treatment is more effective when detected early. To implement this, HIV tests should be offered regularly by health care providers so that more infected people can become aware of their condition and the early opportunistic infections can be treated.

3. The Commission recommends easily accessible, voluntary testing for the protection of those infected as well as those not infected.

4. HIV infections should be treated as a disability under federal and state laws in both the public and private sectors. Infected persons should be allowed and encouraged to continue with normal activities such as school and work, and they should remain in their own homes as long as they are able.

5. The Commission urges stronger protection of the privacy of those with HIV, with penalties for violation of confidentiality, but with a list of clearly defined exceptions.

6. Immediate preventive measures include the institution of nationwide, confidential partner notification. This system would notify those intimate (having sexual relations) with persons carrying sexually transmitted diseases, including HIV. In addition, all health care facilities should notify all those who received blood transfusions since 1978 that they may have been exposed to HIV and may require testing and counseling.

7. Prevention and treatment of drug abuse must become a national priority. Not only should law enforcement efforts to interrupt the drug supply be increased, but it must be coupled with a broadly expanded treatment capacity.

8. Illegal drug and alcohol use help increase the spread of HIV by impairing judgment and depressing the immune system. Those involved in stopping the spread of HIV should bear this in mind. Education for all citizens, especially school children, adolescents, and minorities is essential.

9. The nursing shortage must be addressed to provide adequate care for all areas of society, as well as those greatly affected by HIV infection. One way would be to offer immediate scholarship and loan programs.

10. The National Health Service Corps, which places health care professionals in underserved areas and is scheduled for termination, should not only be extended, but expanded.

11. Greater flexibility should be given to the National Institutes of Health by removing liability obstacles so that its research goals can be achieved. Clinical trials should be expanded to include a broader base of the infected population.

12.   The nation should move toward an organized system of care for infected individuals, in order to control costs and provide quality care, with case management as a principal tool.

13.   Concerns of health care workers need to be better addressed by all levels of government. These workers, and all who are involved in the health care delivery system, should have complete information about HIV, adequate protective materials, and a safe working environment.

14.   The Food and Drug Administration should place top priority on new, quicker HIV detection tests in order to assure the safety of the nation's blood supply, as well as continued research into further protecting the blood supply.

15.   Transfusions of one's own blood should be used whenever possible. Health care facilities need to aggressively train their staff to inform patients of autologous (using your own blood) transfusions as well as of the risks involved with transfusion.

16.   Comprehensive education programs in all our schools, appropriate for age and grade, should be a national priority.

17.   The problems of the disadvantaged, particularly HIV-infected "boarder babies", draw attention to the critical need for foster care. Without attention to the disadvantaged, there will be large increases in both pediatric and drug-related HIV disease.

18.   The problems of teens, especially runaways, who are at an increased risk for HIV infection, should be aggressively addressed. Inaccurate and misleading statements suggesting that HIV cannot be spread through heterosexual activity needs to be clarified in light of the spread within that community.

19.   Several ethical considerations and responsibilities have become most important as a result of the HIV epidemic. First, those who are HIV-infected have a responsibility not to infect others. Second, the health care community has a responsibility to offer care to all HIV-infected persons.   Third, all citizens have a responsibility to treat HIV-infected persons with respect and compassion.

20.   The U.S. should encourage and assist with international efforts to stop the spread of HIV infection through our research community and our contribution to the World Health Organization and the Global Programme on AIDS.

The Commission proposed a budget of $1,997.5 billion greater than the federal government appropriated for FY88. It also called for $1,102.5 billion from the states, for a total budget of $3,100 billion. The largest single allocation was for drug abuse treatment and prevention.

BUDGET ESTIMATES FOR FINAL REPORT RECOMMENDATIONS

(In millions)

	Total Federal dollars over FY 88 appropriated	Total State	Total
Prevention and education	200	100	300
Incidence and prevalence	50		50
Drug abuse	924.5	750	1,674.5
International	25		25
Finance	200	200	400
Patient care	247.5	52.5	300
Research	300		300
Societal	50.5		50.5
Total	1,997.5	1,102.5	3,100

These are the estimated low end (start-up funding) cost estimates for the recommendations.

Source: Report of the Presidential Commission on the Human Immunodeficiency Virus Epidemic, (WDC, 1988)

APPENDIX I - AIDS INFORMATION LIST

American Red Cross
AIDS Education Office
1730 D Street NW
Washington, DC 20006
(202) 737-8300

BEBASHI
1319 Locust St.
Philadelphia, PA 19107
(215) 546-4140

Centers for Disease Control
Office of Public Inquiries
Building 1, Room B-63
1600 Clifton Road
Atlanta, GA 30333
(404) 329-2891

HERO
101 West Read St., Suite 812
Baltimore, MD 21201
(301) 685-1180

Hispanic AIDS Forum
140 West 22 St., Suite 301
New York, NY 10011
(212) 463-8264

The Kupona Network
4611 South Ellis
Chicago, IL 60653
(312) 536-3000

Minority AIDS Project
5882 West Pico Blvd., Suite 210
Los Angeles, CA 90019
(213) 936-4949

Minority Task Force on AIDS
92 St. Nicholas Ave., Suite 1B
New York, NY 10026
(212) 749-2816

Mothers of AIDS Patients (MAP)
4103 10th Avenue
San Diego, CA 92103
(619) 293-3985

National AIDS Network
729 Eighth Street NE, Suite 300
Washington, DC 20003
(202) 293-2437

National Association of
People With AIDS
2025 I Street NW, Suite 415
Washington, DC 20006
(202) 429-2856

National Council of Churches/
AIDS Task Force
475 Riverside Drive, Room 572
New York, NY 10115
(212) 219-8180

National Native American
Prevention Center on AIDS
5266 Boyd Ave.
Oakland, CA 94618
(415) 654-2093

National Minority AIDS Council
714 G Street SE
Washington, DC 20035
(202) 544-1076

San Francisco Black Coalition on AIDS
URSA Institute
185 Berry St., #6600
San Francisco, CA 94107
(415) 822-7228

U.S. Public Health Service
Public Affairs Office
Hubert H. Humphrey Bldg.,Rm. 725-H
200 Independence Avenue SW
Washington, DC 20201
(202) 472-4248

NATIONAL TOLL- FREE HOTLINES

Public Health Service
National AIDS Hotline

(800) 342-AIDS (Recording)
(800) 342-7514 (Answers to specific
questions)

National Sexually Transmitted
Diseases Hotline/American
Social Health Association

(800) 227-8922

National Gay Task Force
AIDS Information Hotline

(800) 221-7044
(212) 806-6016 (in New York State)

Nov. 30 — CDC reports 6,993 AIDS cases; 3,342 known dead (48 percent)

<u>1985</u>

Jan. 8 — WHO reports 559 AIDS cases in 10 European countries.

Mar. 22 — WHO reports 762 AIDS cases in 17 European countries.

May 10 — As of April 30, CDC reports 10,000 AIDS cases; 4,942 are known dead (49 percent of the adults and 69 percent of the children).

May 24 — U.S. Public Health Service recommends testing all donated blood, organs, tissues, and semen for AIDS virus.

Aug. 2 — WHO reports 940 cases in 17 European countries.

Aug. 23 — Two Gallup polls reveal that 95 percent of the U.S. population has heard about AIDS.

Aug. 30 — CDC issues recommendations for the education and foster care of AIDS-infected children.

Sept. 27 — WHO reports 1,226 AIDS cases in 17 European Countries.

Oct. 25 — International Conference of AIDS held in Paris.

Nov. 15 — CDC issues recommendations for transmitting AIDS virus in the workplace.

<u>1986</u>

Jan. 17 — CDC reports 16,458 AIDS patients; 8,361 known dead, (51 percent of adults and 59 percent the children).

Jan. 24 — WHO reports 1,573 AIDS cases in 21 European countries.

Feb. 7 — Possible impact of AIDS virus on tuberculosis cases in 1895.

Mar. 14 — CDC issues recommendations to reduce sexual and drug-related transmission of AIDS virus.

Mar. 28 — National Institute of Justice reports 455 AIDS cases in the state/federal correctional system and 311 in the city/county system.

July 4 — A Dept. of Defense testing of 308,076 applicants for military service found 1.5 per 1,000 recruit applicants showed positive for AIDS virus.

Oct. 24 — Of the 24,567 AIDS cases, 6,192 (25 percent) were black and 3,488 (14 percent) were Hispanic.

Oct. 31 — As of Sept. 15, 238 hemophilia-associated AIDS cases have been reported.

Dec. 12 — CDC reports 28,089 AIDS cases(27,704 adults and 394 children); 15,757 are known dead (56 percent of adults and 61% of children). Over 79 percent of those diagnosed before January 1985 are known dead.

<u>1987</u>

Mar. 20 — AIDS virus reported among multiply-transfused leukemia patients in New York City.

May 22 — Six health care workers who provided care to AIDS (HIV infected) patients and denied other risk factors have been reported with HIV infection.

Dec. 18 — Over 46,00 cases of AIDS has been reported to CDC since 1981.

<u>1988</u>

Jan. 29 — First reported case of (HIV-2) in the U.S. was reported in a West African woman.

Jan. 29 — CDC issues guidelines for effective school health education to prevent spread of AIDS.

Feb. 5 — CDC and FDA (Food and Drug Administration) issue recommendations regarding storage and use of semen, organs and tissues.

June 27 — CDC reports 65,780 cases of AIDS since 1981, 64,731 adults and 1,049 children. Of these 37,195 persons are known dead, 36,590 adults and 605 children.

CHRONOLOGY OF AIDS (From the Centers for Disease Control - Morbidity and Mortality Weekly Reports)

1981

June 5 — Pneumocystis pneumonia diagnosed in 5 homosexual men in Los Angles.

July 3 — Twenty-six cases of Kaposi's sarcoma and 10 additional cases of Pneumocystis pneumonia diagnosed in homosexual men in New York City and California.

Aug. 28 — Seventy additional cases of Kaposi's sarcoma and Pneumocystis pneumonia reported among homosexual men.

1982

May 21 — Fifty-seven cases of persistent, generalized lymphadenopathy among homosexual males in New York City and San Francisco.

June 4 — Four cases of diffuse, undifferentiated non-Hodgkins lymphoma (DONHL) among homosexual males in San Francisco.

June 18 — Cluster of Kaposi's and Pneumocystis carinii pneumonia among previously healthy homosexual males in Los Angles and Orange County.

July 9 — Nineteen cases of opportunistic infections and Kaposi's sarcoma among Haitians in the U.S. (Miami, FL).

July 16 — Three cases of Pneumocystis carinii among hemophilia A patients in Westchester County, NY; Denver, CO, and northeastern Ohio.

Sept. 24 — Between June 1, 1981 and September 15, 1982 CDC reports 593 cases of Acquired Immune Deficiency Syndrome (AIDS), and 243 deaths (41 percent of the total cases).

Dec. 10 — Four additional hemophilia A patients with AIDS in Alabama, Pennsylvania, Ohio, and Missouri.

Dec. 10 — Possible transfusion-associated AIDS in 20 month old infant in San Francisco area.

Dec. 17 — Unexplained immunodeficiency and opportunistic infections in 4 infants in New York, New Jersey and California.

1983

Jan. 7 — Immunodeficiency in 2 female sexual partners of male with AIDS in New York.

Jan. 7 — New York and New Jersey report 16 prison inmates with AIDS.

May 13 — Human T-cell leukemia virus infection in several AIDS patients.

June 24 — As of June 20, 1983, there were 1,641 cases of AIDS reported; 644 are known dead (38 percent).

Aug. 5 — As of August 1, there were 1,972 cases of AIDS reported; 759 known dead (38 percent).

Sept. 2 — CDC publishes precautions for health-care workers and allied professionals.

Sept. 9 — CDC reports 2,259 AIDS cases; 917 known dead (41 percent).

Nov. 25 — World Health Organization (WHO) reports 267 European AIDS cases.

Nov. 25 — Canada reports 51 cases of AIDS.

Dec. 2 — CDC reports a total of 21 AIDS cases among hemophilia patients.

1984

Jan. 6 — As of Dec. 19, 1983, CDC reports 3,000 AIDS cases; 1,283 known dead (43 percent).

June 22 — As of June 18, 1983, CDC reports 4,918 AIDS cases; 2,221 known dead (45 percent). More than 76 percent of those diagnosed before July 1892 are dead.

Aug. 3 — International Conference on AIDS meets in Atlanta.

Oct. 26 — A total of 52 hemophilia patients have been diagnosed with AIDS.

Nov. 2 — WHO reports 420 AIDS cases in 10 European countries.

monoclonal derived from a single cell.

morbidity frequency of disease occurrence in proportion to the population.

mortality frequency of number of deaths in proportion to the population.

myelopathy pathological changes in the bone marrow.

NDA New Drug Application. After clinical trials are completed, an NDA is filed with the Food and Drug Administration so that the drug may be placed in the market.

oncovirus sub-family of retroviruses that includes tumor-causing agents.

opportunistic infection an infection caused by an organism that rarely causes disease in persons with normal immune systems but attacks immunosuppressed patients. Infections common in patients with AIDS include toxoplasmosis, *pneumocystis carinii* pneumonia, cytomegalovirus, and tuberculosis.

orphan drugs drugs designated for use in diseases with annual patient incidence of 200,000 or less, or for which the company is not expected to be able to make a profit. Tax benefits and market exclusivity accompany orphan drug status.

parenteral taken into the body other than through the digestive tract, as by intravenous or intramuscular injection.

pathogenesis the development of morbid conditions or of disease, more specifically, the cellular events and reactions and other mechanisms occurring in the development of disease.

perinatal occurring near the time of birth.

peripheral neuropathies functional disturbances and/or changes in the peripheral nervous system.

persistent generalized lymphadenopathy (PGL) a condition characterized by swollen glands that remain enlarged despite the absence of known current illness or drug use.

pharmacology science which deals with the study of the action of drugs on living systems.

placebo an inactive substance used as a control in an experiment.

placebo controlled trials clinical trials in which patients are randomized to one treatment group or another. One group of the trial participants receive the study drug and the other half receive a placebo. In double blind studies, neither the patient nor the physician knows if the patient is getting the drug or the placebo. This is done to eliminate the "placebo effect," the early positive response of almost all patients to receiving any therapy.

***pneumocystis carinii* pneumonia** opportunistic infection most frequently diagnosed in patients with AIDS. Caused by a parasite commonly present in the normal population, *pneumocystis carinii* infection is life-threatening in immunosuppressed patients.

polyclonal derived from different cells.

principal investigator lead scientist running a study or lead doctor running a clinical trial.

psychobiology interactions between body and mind in the formation and functioning of personality.

P-3 biosafety level applicable to clinical, diagnostic, teaching, research, or production facilities in which work is done with agents which may cause serious or potentially lethal reactions as a result of exposure by inhalation. Practically, there must be special airflows and filters, an antechamber with sink, protective garments must always be worn, and nothing may be taken out of the room without being sterilized.

reagent substance used in a chemical reaction to detect, examine, measure, or produce other substances. In virology, strains of HIV are reagents.

recombinant DNA DNA prepared through laboratory manipulation in which genes from one species of an organism are transplanted or spliced to another organism.

retrovirus one of a group of viruses that have RNA as their genetic code and have the ability to copy that RNA into DNA and incorporate it into an infected cell.

reverse transcriptase an enzyme produced by retroviruses that allows them to produce a DNA copy of their RNA. This is the first step in their natural cycle of reproduction.

RNA (ribonucleic acid) basic genetic material. A nucleic acid associated with the control of chemical activities inside a cell.

sero- prefix referring to blood serum.

seroconversion the initial development of antibodies specific to blood serum.

serologic pertaining to blood serum.

seropositive condition in which antibodies to a specific antigen are found in the blood.

seroprevalence prevalence based on blood serum tests.

serostatus condition of the blood -- infected or uninfected.

shooting gallery location where drug addicts meet to "shoot" intravenous drugs, often sharing needles.

STDs sexually transmitted diseases.

surveillance process of monitoring public health conditions such as epidemics. Passive surveillance monitors conditions through the receipt of reports; active surveillance employs investigative techniques.

syndrome pattern of symptoms and signs, appearing one by one or simultaneously that together characterize a particular disease or disorder.

T-cell cell that matures in the thymus gland. T-lymphocytes are found primarily in the blood, lymph, and lymphoid organs. Subsets of T-cells have a variety of specialized functions within the immune system.

T4 cell count measure of the state of the immune system based on the number of T4 lymphocytes present in the blood.

treatment use regulations Also: compassionate use. Process by which a drug company applies to the Food and Drug Administration, in special cases, to distribute drugs to the desperately ill even though the drug has not been approved for use outside a clinical trial. In some cases, this also applies to drugs that have been approved for use but not for the disease for which it is being requested. A change in the rules in June 1987 allowed for the release of such drugs earlier than usual for AIDS, but to date, only one has been so used.

virology study of viruses and virus diseases.

Western blot blood test that involves the identification of antibodies against specific protein molecules. This test is more specific than the ELISA test in detecting antibodies to HIV in blood samples. It is used as a confirmatory test for positive ELISA samples. The Western blot requires more sophisticated lab technique than the ELISA and is more expensive.

GLOSSARY

affective pertaining to a feeling or mental state.

AIDS Treatment Evaluation Unit (ATEU) original name of the AIDS Clinical Trial Groups, established by National Institute of Allergy and Infectious Diseases to test new AIDS-related drugs.

AIDS Clinical Trial Group (ACTG) experimental drug testing system administrated by National Institute of Allergy and Infectious Diseases. Also, one of the 35 medical centers in the group.

animal models trials done in animals prior to human studies. For example, tests of various substances in standardized genetic strains of mice or the tests of HIV vaccine in chimpanzees.

antibody a molecule produced in response to antigen which has the particular property of combining specifically with the antigen which induced its formation.

antigen a molecule which induces the formation of an antibody.

aseptic meningitis inflammation of the membranes that envelop the brain and spinal column caused by a viral agent.

autologous transfusion blood transfusion in which the patient receives his or her own blood.

basic research research in the basic or pure sciences. Not product-oriented.

candidiasis yeastlike fungus infection. A common opportunistic infection.

clinical trials studies in human subjects.

co-factors those factors which can influence an individual's likelihood of becoming ill or influence the progression of disease. Commonly cited HIV-related co-factors include a history of intravenous drug abuse, and presence or history of sexually transmitted diseases or other immunocompromising conditions.

cohort studies studies that follow groups of similar individuals over time, noting who develops a disease and who does not, and comparing these two groups at the end of the study to determine co-factors and other elements that may influence outcome. Cohort studies of gay men in San Francisco have determined that behavior modification can influence incidence of HIV infection, and reduce the number of new cases.

crystallography the study of crystal structure. Used to study the structure of crystallized viruses.

cytomegalovirus one of a group of herpes viruses that infect man, monkeys, and rodents.

dementia general designation for mental deterioration.

DNA (deoxyribonucleic acid) basic genetic material. A nucleic acid found chiefly in the nucleus of living cells that is responsible for transmitting hereditary characteristics.

double blind trials see placebo controlled trials.

ELISA acronym for "enzyme-linked immunosorbent assay," a test used to detect antibodies against HIV.

epidemiology study of the relationships of the various factors determining the frequency and distribution of diseases in a human environment.

etiology study of the factors that cause disease.

genome the genetic "endowment" of an organism. A complete set of chromosomes.

GP 120 glycoprotein on the surface of HIV and a target for several potential vaccines.

Hodgkin's disease a chronic progressive disease of unknown etiology that is characterized by inflammatory enlargement of the lymph nodes, spleen, and often liver and kidneys.

hospice establishment or program which cares for the physical and emotional needs of terminally ill patients.

HTLV human T-cell lymphotropic virus. This is the family of viruses to which HIV belongs.

immunology the medical study of the immune system.

immunomodulators drugs which alter the state of immune system, usually to improve response.

immunosuppression artificial prevention or diminution of the immune response.

in vitro "in glass", observable in a test tube.

IND (investigational new drug) status of a drug after approval for use in clinical trials but before approval for marketing.

institutional review board (IRB) committee within a hospital or other institution through which all new research protocols and projects must pass. IRBs are comprised of physician members of each medical service, nurses, administrators, and patient representatives. They check to see consent forms are properly worded, all procedures are properly followed, etc.

intervention (in behavior modification research) those techniques or devices by which one behavior is interrupted and another, presumably healthier, behavior is instituted.

Kaposi's sarcoma a cancer or tumor of the blood and/or lymphatic vessel walls. It is a common opportunistic infection in HIV infection.

LAV (lymphadenopathy-associated virus) the name given by French researchers to the first reported isolate of the retrovirus now known to cause AIDS.

lentivirus a virus that can cross the blood/brain barrier, destroy brain tissue, and remain in the body in a chronic sub-clinical state for long periods. HIV is a lentivirus that causes forms of mental incapacity in an estimated 70 to 80 percent of patients, and end-stage dementia in many. Lentiviruses persist in the body by evading natural defense mechanisms. In animals, the chronic state is common. In this state, animals infected with a lentivirus are "carriers" and may not get sick themselves for a long time, but can transmit the virus to other animals.

look-back program program that attempts to identify recipients of blood from a donor who is later found to be HIV antibody positive.

lymphadenopathy disease of the lymph nodes.

lymphocyte white blood cells, some of which are involved in the immune response.

lymphoma any of the various cancers of the lymphoid tissue.

magic bullet in theory, a single drug that can knock out a particular malignant cell or other disorder without any toxicity.

microbiology science which deals with the study of microorganisms, including bacte-

INDEX